Praise

"In her latest book, *Deeper Days*, author and yogi master Andrea L. Wehlann has created a daily inspirational book that will motivate you to delve deeper into your yoga practise. This book is full of enlightened words to incorporate into your everyday life as well as expanding your knowledge of the history and deeper meanings of yoga. As a Doctor of Chiropractic, I find yoga the perfect supplement to reduce stress, improve balance and body strength for anyone seeking a wellness lifestyle. I will recommend this book to my patients, whether they are beginners or advanced yogis, to help with their healing journey."
Dr. Amber Gardiner, Grimbsy, Ontario

"The great yogic sage Patanjali taught us that daily consistency of practice is the key to living life in our true state—pure unbounded consciousness. But how do we get there? In *Deeper Days*, Andrea gives us the foundation, the blueprint, and the fuel to show up each day and authentically live the teachings. Through daily inquiry and practice of the eight limbs, we are lovingly guided on a year-long journey of expansion & personal transformation. This book is a precious gift to every yogi looking to shift your life from where you are to where you'd like to be."
davidji, Author of *Sacred Powers: The Five Secrets to Awakening Transformation*

"This tome celebrates the blessed union of the mind + body + spirit through daily introspection. Read to immerse yourself in the energy of the mindful messages that inspire all sentient beings. Harness the genuine warmth as you feel the love resonates from the pages."
Tiffany L. Gallagher, Ph.D., Professor, Department of Educational Studies & Director, Brock Learning Lab

Deeper Days

365 Yoga-spirations for Inner Calm Amidst Chaos

By Andrea L. Wehlann

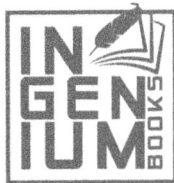

INGENIUM BOOKS

ISBNs
eBook: 978-1-990688-03-4
paperback: 978-1-990688-02-7

Editing by Marie Beswick Arthur
Book cover design by Jessica Bell
Book formatting by Amie McCracken

Nikola Rocco, Luka Andrija, Andreas Milan, Brad, Potato and 7 Stars

Opening and Circling

It takes approximately 365 days for Earth to complete one orbit around the Sun. In this book, I hold space for your own magnificent journey to unfold—for you to experience that you are creation itself.

I offer a trail of my footprints as tracks on a path of living omnipresence.

We are interconnected in possibility, moving through the world with love as the quality of awareness and the driving force behind our actions.

In the same way a cool river flows to an open sea, your life and your yoga practice are seamless continuities of each other. You are the current you've been waiting for.

Deeper Days encourages an open message of daily self-inquiry. Through yoga the practices of meditation, postures, and breathing techniques may sometimes feel separate from daily life. This book has been designed to banish dualities, burn the illusion of a separate self into the alchemical fires of transmutation, clarifying destiny of dwelling in possibility, so that every action becomes an expression of yoga, love, and you.

How To Use This Book

Whether you are a yoga teacher, yoga student, or both, I honour your intentions as you celebrate this path of all those masters whose energy surrounds us. It's as simple as turning a page each day, as adventurous as you choose to make it, and deeper than any ocean.

Ideally, as you read, and reflect, notice what arises: kiss the page, bless the statement, trace the words with your fingertips—even write it out—close your eyes, imagine an ancient sage speaking its energy through you. Feel that message in your heart—you choose how to take it in. I encourage you to keep it with you as you move through your day.

I have structured the daily messages on the eight limbs of yoga, and provided more detail about them to help you experience the bliss of *Deeper Days*.

Simplicity is love, joy, peace, and divine grace. Simplicity is expressed in this book by numbering the days of your orbit, not by identifying them with a specific day within a specific month. Your year begins on DAY 1, or whichever number resonates with you in the present. Be gentle with yourself—if you miss a day, let it go, move on. Every page is a fresh start—we forget and remember again and forget again. This is your unique trip around the sun.

Within these days you'll align to frequencies that will resonate so strongly for you that you do a deeper dive, choose to engage in and with different actions, people, or places. The power of love—my love for you—exists in the now, within each word of every entry.

As evolving sentient spirits expressing or embodying yoga and sharing its magnificence, may you be supported for deeper days on the yoga mat and beyond. When you are ready to dig further into your unique expression of even deeper days, consider purchasing the Deeper Days Companion Journal, available here: ingeniumbooks.com/DeeperDaysJournal

The Sacred Responsibility: Guiding and Inspiring

In yoga instructor training, the concept of understanding union with reality often features in the classes—becoming one with the self. Long-time students of yoga hear this message too. They ways of guiding and teaching have changed as societies developed. As East met the West, branches of practices have been branded, and yoga posture images sensationalized through media and marketing. Yet yoga's essence must remain as intended: oneness. Oneness is becoming "one" with whatever arises, open to shifts, one with whatever is flowing in life. We don't do oneness, we be oneness. There is nothing to "do" because everything is already connected.

Patañjali was a sage in ancient India who has been credited with a number of Sanskrit works. Born 200 years BCE, and passing in 150 BCE, the works considered to be his greatest are the Yoga Sutras which are contained in a classical yoga text.

Patañjali said:

> *"Yoga is the settling of the mind into silence.*
> *When the mind has settled,*
> *we are established in our essential nature,*
> *which is unbounded Consciousness.*
> *Our essential nature is usually overshadowed by the activity of the mind."*

How beautiful and refreshing is that?

What a divine river is yoga—not even a sense of ego on the riverbanks—only pure clarity that flows its soulful current between the heart and the brain, the hands and feet, blurring the lines between where the skin ends and spirit continues, wrapping around mountains, rolling through cities, swirling and living.

Patañjali explains there are eight limbs of yoga—eight modes—which can be done separately but are done together to attain moksha… emancipation (meaning to come into your own truthful space and recognize your essence).

The eight limbs of yoga are:

1. Yama (guidelines/ethics)
2. Niyama (observances)
3. Asana (yoga postures)
4. Pranayama (breath control)
5. Pratyahara (withdrawal of the senses)
6. Dharana (concentration)
7. Dhyana (meditation), and
8. Samadhi (absorption).

The first six are practices. The last two are things that happen to us (because of doing the first six).

The cultural impressions we consume often portray yoga as stretching. Devoted teachers and students of yoga understand that physical posture is a part of a whole of the eight limbs of yoga. Yoga trends for wellness are helpful gateways to liberating the mind from stuck patterns that cause disease and poor health, including negative self-talk. The essence of yoga, however, is whatever word you use for mindfulness—nature, love, light, universe. Wherever you are, whatever you believe, start there. This is the essence of the Zen saying: start where you are.

Yoga's essence is not the latest mat or popular outfit. Essence is within you: formless and ethereal.

I teach my students that yoga is a breathing practice. I use breath as an object of meditation and focus. It brings us closer to our essence. Returning to the breath in this way silences some of the static of the mind.

Breath bridges the physical and spiritual worlds.

Patañjali's words are timeless, and represent formlessness.

Patañjali outlines a framework for yoga practice made up of eight different limbs that coexist—they are essential elements on the journey of the self, through the self, to the self. Yes, that journey of self-realization. Breathing is a way into the self. That journey is an enlightening one. No wonder Marianne Williamson says that we are not afraid of the dark and that, instead, we are afraid of the light.

The Truth and Sutras

Sutras, literally, refer to a collection of aphorisms—which are like short sayings of truths—in a kind of manual of ancient times. They are basically a genre of ancient texts found in Hinduism, Buddhism, and Jainism.

The Yoga Sutras of Patañjali, written in Sanskrit, focus on the theory and practice of yoga. The sutras are like the threads that weave cloth together. They allow for the creation of consciousness which is needed to live a life of less suffering and more pleasantness and provide a way to freedom from thought patterns. They support creativity and help us to break harmful patterns we carry in our bodies.

We are an intricate design of super-consciousness. As we evolved—as a people, within cultures—we suffered from the outcomes our own intelligence. If we use the sutras and eight limbs as a guide to the inner-workings of the mind, we can have a life free from thoughts and stories that are no longer useful. We can let go of what no longer serves us. We can celebrate an attitude of kindness and gratitude.

The universe is waiting for us. We create the journey of the self, through the self, to the self. We enhance that journey by adding daily acts of kindness, gratitude lists, and accessing reminders like the ones in this book. I say to my students, "Use the breath to remember." Now I say to you, "Breathe through the turning of these pages."

The 1st Limb: Yama (Ethics)

There is no yoga without ethics. Yamas create self-discipline for a chaotic mind. If we do not set parameters for what we do, then there is no meaning to what we do.

While deep into a yoga ethics course with my Zen Buddhist teacher, I believed I was nonviolent. But with self-inquiry practice, I realized that many of my good intentions were stories I created to uphold my nonviolent belief.

I wrote out the ways I contribute to harm. I went deep.

This is what embodying an ethic in simple terms in daily life looks like: I used to take an interest in the cheap celebrity magazines at the grocery checkouts. In applying this ethic I realized that by buying a magazine with a picture of Princess Diana on the cover, for example, I was contributing to the violence perpetrated by the paparazzi which ultimately may have contributed to her death. I stopped buying those magazines.

The 2ⁿᵈ Limb: Niyama (Self-Observances/Discipline)

Niyama is the coming to understand the self. It's our observances, awareness, and taking note of the little things we do. It is a practice to evaluate our conduct—for example, the way we turn on and off water (softly, conservation-mindedly), the way we prepare our meals, the way we smile and wave. The niyama is mindfulness and awareness. When individuals are mindful, they are never going to be manipulative—their intent is pure. Becoming mindful means letting go of the ego.

The 3ʳᵈ Limb: Asana (Physical Postures)

The asanas are physical forms; this is where we're forming shapes with our body. This is what many people think yoga is.

When we do positions, the movement awakens the body and transforms it into an expression of our physical essence.

The 4ᵗʰ Limb: Pranayama (Breath Control)

Pranayama is controlled breathing… remember the first six of the eight limbs are what we do. Pranayama is flowing and filling the body with life-energy (oxygen) and all things in the air.

When we are filled with energy, we can recognize the body is a tool; it's not who we permanently are. The breath reminds us of the gift of refreshing our nervous system and supporting our mindfully mindless practice.

The 5ᵗʰ Limb: Pratyahara (Withdrawal of Senses)

Pratyahara is one of the hardest things to do. It entails removing things that we believe to be pleasurable. Note the "believe to be." So set in our ways are we that we covet things, develop clutter (and call it a collection), indulge in distractions that include the consumption of certain food and drink, utter hurtful words— all in the name of feeling superior.

Pratyahara is an inside job—recognizing what doesn't serve us, freeing ourselves from that which doesn't. Successfully achieving pratyahara is to re-evaluate our reliance on externally-motivated happiness.

The 6th Limb: Dharana (Concentration)

Dharana means pure focus, a single track in the mind that discounts multi-tasking. It is a state of focussing on one thing. When we practice dharana, our ability to concentrate is strengthened. There becomes less identification with and less attachment to storytelling. We achieve one pure truth. In this way we are calm, become more confident, and free ourselves from chaos.

The 7th Limb: Dhyana (Meditation)

We keep our focus for a longer period, awareness of what arises in the present moment. The space of meditation is as close to thoughtlessness as we can get. An isolation—thoughtlessness being the ultimate nature, simplicity, creativity, and process to reach freedom within pure consciousness.

The 8th Limb: Samadhi (Peace)

The eighth limb is experiencing oneness with reality. The realization of interconnection, wholeness, and our infinite potential.

Experiential observation: you can't explain to someone how samadhi feels any more than you can the subtleties of the taste of a fresh peach. One simply experiences it. This state is also referred to as bliss or ecstasy. Similar to the arising of insight in meditation, it is experiential.

Remember: limbs one to six are things we do through conscious decision—actions we consciously decide to take. The seventh and eighth we experience because of practicing one through six. As a garden, tending the soil and planting seeds is limbs one to six. Limbs seven and eight are the luscious fruits which appear because of our nurturing.

As you ready yourself to dive into deeper days, which I've organized thematically into the eight limbs, each of the sets of days begins with a deeper exploration of the associated limb.

Yama: The 1st Limb

"Something amazing happens when we surrender and just love. We melt into another world, a realm of power already within us. The world changes when we change. The world softens when we soften. The world loves us when we choose to love the world."
MARIANNE WILLIAMSON, *A WOMAN'S WORTH*

Yamas are moral, ethical, and spiritual standards a person acquires to balance their health and well-being. The yama's five characteristics are contained in our actions, words, and thoughts.

1. Ahimsa: Nonviolence

Ahimsa is to not cause harm to ourselves or any other living being. Ahimsa is compassion towards all. Apply it to your life by asking yourself whether your thoughts, actions, and behaviour are facilitating growth within you and others around you. Are you positively contributing to your relationships? Observe how you interact with, and relate to, others—is harm present? Is there space for you to show compassion?

2. Satya: Honesty

Satya is a dedication to being as honest as you can be. The healthiest version of our being is one who speaks truthfully within our heart to those around us. Honesty can often be a scary thing. For example, we think we may hurt someone by being truthful. Not being truthful can sometimes be much more harmful for us and for our loved ones. Honesty can be expressed with care and compassion. In this way honesty is liberating.

Apply satya to your life by acknowledging what is true for you now. You can then broaden this to a moment-to-moment practice. How do you express yourself honestly? Do you base your truth on someone else's explanation of the truth, or have you experienced it as your own? When you hear gossip, think about whether it is really something you want to communicate forward.

3. Asteya: Non-Stealing

If we obtain something that has not been freely given to us, it can be considered stealing. It does not simply refer to stealing money or possessions from someone. Asteya self-inquiry asks how often we try to steal time from others. Do I attempt to persuade someone to do something they don't freely want to do? Am I seeking someone's attention when they are not willing to give it freely?

Non-stealing also means cultivating a feeling of abundance within. It is realizing we do not lack anything, rather we have everything. We can be grateful for the things we have instead of trying to take what is not naturally ours.

Apply asteya to your life by observing your feelings. Do you feel you are bathing in abundance, or are you constantly looking for something extra to satisfy you and make you happy? Do you demand time and attention from others? Do you let others steal your time and attention?

4. Brahmacharya: Sexual Energy

What brahmacharya means is to be aware of how we use our sexual energy. All yamas aim to free us from serving our egoic cravings and desires so that we may open to something greater.

When we attune to sexual energy as a creative current flowing within us, experiences can be what they can be at best, intimate expressions of love, perhaps even between two people, this can be a great addition to our spiritual journey.

Apply brahmacharya to your life by considering what you spend your creative and sexual energy on. Notice habits of clinging and attachments, as these tend to entangle and block the flow of brahmacharya. Do your habits allow or repress its natural flow? Without attachment to stories and circumstances, there can be wisdom in our actions. Can you allow this energy to open beyond the ego and into the ethereal dimensions of being?

5. Aparigraha: Non-Coveting

Holding on to things does not allow us to be free. Aparigraha is a deep letting go of the need to hold onto material items, certain ideas, concepts about life, and events. It even involves relinquishing those holding-on patterns within personality—the stories, feelings, beliefs we accumulate from the outside world. At some point, with yoga, we reach for something greater than the repetition of our cycles of satisfaction and dissatisfaction. Aparigraha reminds nothing belongs to us in the first place. We can be present in each moment authentically meeting life as it is happening now.

When we understand life is in constant change, we change and can responsibly redirect our energies to support and develop with it, as a practice. We can come back to the breath and feel sensations in the body, which is always in the present moment, and we can trust in the universe that we have all we need to respond skillfully to situations.

Apply aparigraha to your life by inquiring what you need to be you. What can you renounce? Can you trust life to give you what you need without holding onto anything?

Practicing the yamas can balance our mental, physical, and spiritual energies. They are the perfect building blocks for a long-lasting, peaceful relationship with our selves, and those around us.

The Yama Days

Day 1
Personally Peaceable

Yoga is a path. The first step on that path is to do no harm—a nonviolent step. Nonviolence to others, the earth, and ourselves.

We can all become more peaceable humans. We can ask ourselves: "How do I contribute to harm?"

By paying attention to and studying the self, we become more mindful of the things we do that cause harm and, as a result, become closer to the process of yoking (uniting) with the true self.

Yoga is unity of mental and physical energies.

yoga, or to yoke, means to unite

Day 2
Awareness

A bodhisattva in Buddhism is one who seeks awakening. This begins with a commitment to practicing five precepts.

1. Ahimsa: Nonviolence
2. Satya: Honesty
3. Asteya: Nongreed, not taking what is freely given
4. Brahmachary: Sexual Energy
5. Aparigraha: Nonacquisitiveness

The release of acquisitiveness (letting go of needing to have and collect posessions), reminding us nothing actually belongs to us in the first place.

Can you commit to and embrace the five precepts as new codes of conduct? How do you feel about each precept in relation to your current relationships?

Which precepts are prevalent in your life?

awareness is growth

Day 3
Perfectly Imperfect Relationships

Relationships reflect our consciousness—our energy, vibration, spirit.

Each relationship can teach, assist, and guide us to become a better human being.

Relationships bring great pleasure and pain. Neither can be avoided.

In knowing pleasure and pain flow together, can you open to feeling these as processes flowing within you? Can you spend less time in pain knowing pleasure is also rising? Can you let go of pleasure-seeking knowing pain is inevitable? Can you notice the cycles of pain and pleasure through the day?

trust in the fluid nature
of pleasure and pain

Day 4
Enter Within, Go Without

Western cultures have conditioned us to look outside ourselves for satisfaction, to reward achievements, and seek certain worldly ideals.

Have you noticed, through your experiences, that you never quite get there? Have you noticed that it always seems something else is coming?

When we accept fluidity as life's nature rather than an existence of a destination, our understanding increases to accept we are always in process; we are process.

we are fluid, constantly changing

Day 5
Shifts in Suffering

When we're suffering, we worry. We don't know how to see past the grief. We think happiness was a dream. This is an illusion, created by our family memories about loss, influenced by what we've seen on television and shaped by our faith. When we acknowledge this illusion, we make space for our natural intelligence to flow.

When we suffer less, we see there are things to look forward to. We experience more joy and contentment. Suffering less allows for more laughter and enjoyment of life.

all emotions are meant to flow

Day 6
Impermanence

After experiencing a devastating loss, if one allows themself to feel the legitimate pain the loss brought and does not avoid feeling that pain, things improve.

We wake one morning to find there's something in the day we're looking forward to. Or someone says something funny, and we're surprised to hear our own laugh. Or we find ourselves able to plan things, even if only a trip to the grocery store.

When we're in the middle of the worst of it all, we feel the grieving is going to stay forever, and that happiness is only a dream.

This is only an illusion brought about by the conditions of current life and not having the ability to see past suffering while you're experiencing it.

Have you ever noticed that, somehow, when you look back at being pushed from a job or relationship, that it was a positive?

Just for today, can you embody the words "trust the process"?

nothing is forever,
including the pain of loss

Day 7
Growing Pains

Without uncertainty, we might never grow because we would never be pushed beyond our comfort zones.

Many of us have experienced staying in a soul-sucking job or an unhealthy relationship because the insecurity of leaving the situation created more anxiety than the certainty of staying in the unhappy situation.

A lot of people do not follow their true passions because doing so would seem impractical, or because there is uncertainty associated with following that path.

Where in your life are you staying for comfort, avoiding certainty? Who will you be if you stay?

growth takes place outside
or on the edge of our comfort zone

Day 8
Enriching Life and Loves

Jealousy makes us paranoid and evokes fear that our friends and/or partners will abandon us. This disturbance can cause us to lose peace of mind.

The more possessive we are, the more we drive others away.

Realizing that we all have an infinite capacity for love helps us overcome resentment.

Having passions, finding enjoyment, and celebrating other people, professions, sports, hobbies, or interests does not diminish the love in a relationship. Such expressions enrich life and relationships.

self-trust is self-love

Day 9
Worthy Collaboration

The only thing we can truly rely on is change. Change is inevitable.

We adapt to change or we decay with it.

This is less of a challenge when, in life, we only have ourselves to reconcile with. Relationships act as a mirror. In that way, we are faced with what we need to change within ourselves.

Today, can you accept you are exactly where you need to be? There's nowhere to get to. You are already here.

What does that feel like to say that to yourself? Let the goodness fill your body from head to toe. Accept you are here, right now.

relationships require collaboration,
and adaptation to change

Day 10
The Great Escape

We can feel vulnerable when uncertainty arrives, so we try to escape it any way we can. We make up stories to justify our action or inaction. That kind of story-telling never leads to a solution.

We make ourselves crazy, spinning our minds through the same handful of scenarios we come up with, over and over, never feeling any closer to some resolution.

Stillness is the answer. Can you be still today? Can you notice stillness as an essential element of your nature?

sharing our vulnerability...
opening the door to let people in...
is a loving-self solution

Day 11
The Light in the Dark

Compassionate connections exist when each person in the relationship is accomplished in knowing their own shadow side.

Our shadow is usually unconscious, repressed, containing aspects of ourselves we want to hide. Today, make a list of your shadow qualities. You may experience moments of awakening.

to identify and accept our own darkness
is self-work with a unifying future

Day 12
Our Nature

Interconnectedness is the nature of life.

   Can you apply this to any thoughts of self-harm as now harming the entire web of human existence? The illusion we are separate is the biggest lie. We are essential; we are goodness. We are more than individual; we are a part of a collective whole.

all truthful roads are love

Day 13
Connection

Sometimes, caring about a thing or a person becomes more of an attachment than care.

The Buddha taught that one of the fundamental characteristics of the universe is anicca, meaning that everything changes. We know this is true from our own experience, yet often we hold on to something or someone to make something permanent or secure. We attach and cling by desire and craving. What you cling to can be lost. When we practice letting go, we can begin to experience peace of mind.

letting go is letting love

Day 14
Exploration

Find your perfect self-loving mantras. Mantra is a string of words, or a phrase, or more than one phrase, chanted during meditation. You may already have a saying you tell yourself to stay strong or perhaps a lesson learned you repeat when needed, or a song lyric you love.

A mantra can go beyond a phrase—in this way it can help a person to focus on the positive, stay spiritually strong, even create a new life.

Compose it. Write it down. Hang it up around your space where you will see it often.

your mantra is a force of love you can use
to create the life you're destined to live

Day 15
Onward

When we look for resolution from the outside world, we are seeking, giving away our power.

We can and must embody moving forward regardless of anything in the outside world.

We can forgive ourselves; it is essential to do so over and over.

No one on the outside can ever give to us those things we believe we need. We are born with all we need.

Learn to rely on you. Keep moving forward. Every time you remember your true nature you choose life. Who can you add to a forgiveness list?

today is for you, your heart,
and owning your power

Day 16
Patterns of the Mindful

Certain patterns of thinking are created as we attach stories from memories to thoughts. Excessive tangents and overthinking can drag us down, yet our mind will persist in continuously playing specific thoughts. This happens for us and allows us to create new memories that serve us now.

Who would you be without these thoughts? What skills could you learn to create new patterns that align with the peace and love you are?

change your thoughts,
change your life

Day 17
Ample

Yoga removes layers of societal, ancestral, and cultural accumulations, each revealing the love within us, our nature, wholeness, interconnectedness, connection, unity of mind, body, and soul.

yoga guides us to our infinite potential

Day 18
Karma _Is_ Action

On choosing karma…

Our past memories, or karma, shape our experience of the world. It exists because as sentient human beings, our cells (our body) can hold onto what's already happened. It can only create karma from memories. Therefore, we cannot respond from what we have not experienced.

Awareness is our golden opportunity. Awareness creates space between thought and reaction. With space we can respond more creatively, to act "as if," or "fake it till you make it." Creation of new patterns aligns us with our destiny.

What do you dream of now? How would you feel if you had it now? What do you dream of that is larger than life?

you are a creator

Day 19
Tending the Garden

We look within, and then to the outside world, and we determine our thoughts of separation and the stories we attach to them. This is a point of realization that we must tend to our mind like a garden, pull each weed (a negative thought) by the root or it will grow back. We create conditions in our lives to sustain more loving thoughts by tending to the negative. As seasons change, so do relationships and ideas.

Cultivate love, truth, and all good things. Tend the soil of the mind, water the seeds of wishes and dreams, and take care of what sprouts to help it grow. This is the romance; this is self-love and care.

What are your weeds? Where did they first enter your mind (childhood, TV, family)? Digging deep will allow sun to shine where there once was darkness.

truth transcends and transforms illusion

Day 20
Four for Kindness

In relation to our endeavours to live a spiritual life and make spiritual progress, there are four valuable insights.

1. It is vital to develop positive routines or habits, and to be disciplined.
2. Difficulties will arise… challenges create contrast which creates growth.
3. There is no need to "look" for powerful experiences, only to "see" them.
4. It is fundamental to our spiritual evolution that we hold an attitude of goodwill toward ourselves.

positive routine conditions us
with positive results

Day 21
Becoming

Strong or powerful experiences in meditation are an occasional by-product of the spiritual life. A more significant indicator of an increased pleasantness in life is noticing the kind of person you are becoming.

Have you noticed when you are less reactive and more creative?

How are your relationships?

actions of goodness are
the essence of our nature

Day 22
Kind Voice

Harsh and unkind speech echoes a harsh and unkind atmosphere.

Kind speech creates a loving atmosphere.

By learning to speak in a kind and sensitive manner we create a world around us which is enjoyable to live in. A world where we can relax and be free from the stresses and strains of verbal warfare, crudeness, and malice.

Metta means positive energy and kindness toward others.

Kind speech is the expression of metta and nonviolence, which is the fundamental ethical principle of Buddhism.

kind intention, tone, and words
create a powerful, loving vibration

Day 23
Mercy

Buddhist teachings counsel forgiveness.

In the *Dhammapada* (an anthology of verses attributed to the Buddha), the Buddha gives an instruction that is fierce and compassionate.

> *"If someone has abused you, beat you, robbed you, abandon your thoughts of anger. Soon you will die. Life is too short to live with hatred."*

What some consider small acts of forgiveness, like something domestic in the home, or massive gestures of forgiveness between countries who have warred, the result is the same: freedom from the past.

forgiveness is loving you—forgive often

Day 24
The Four Noble Truths

The heart of the Buddha's teachings lies in the Four Noble Truths, expounded in his very first sermon following his enlightenment.

The first noble truth proclaimed by the Buddha is dukka: Life is suffering, and suffering is a reality.

The second nobel truth, samudaya, is that the cause of this suffering originates in our own minds.

The third noble truth, nirodha, offers hope: Liberation and freedom from suffering is possible.

The fourth noble truth, magga, gives one the method to attain liberation, known to Buddhists as the path of the Middle Way.

there is a middle path

Day 25
The Only Way Out Is In

The Eightfold Path is Buddha's offering to suffer less.
    Right View
    Right Intention
    Right Speech
    Right Action
    Right Effort
    Right Livelihood
    Right Mindfulness
    Right Concentration

the path home is within

Day 26
A Clearer View

To evolve is to keep sight of who we are deep inside—a view of each of us doing the best we can to get over, across, or through challenging times and places.

What is your vision of you at your maximum potential?

we are all-connected,
walking loving steps towards home

Day 27
Perceived Connection

Compassion can be a mixture of desire and attachment. For example, the love a parent has for their child is often linked to the parent's emotional needs, therefore it is not wholly, authentically compassionate.

It can be similar in marriage. The love between husband and wife—especially in the beginning, when one isn't fully aware of the other's character flaws—can be attachment rather than real love.

Our desire from conditioning can be so strong that the person we are attached to only appears good, despite behaving negatively. Our attachment to stories exaggerates qualities. When the dynamic changes, one person is often disappointed. This changes their attitude. This is a sign of love being motivated more from personal need—transactional—rather than authentically intended. To reduce this kind of attachment, we can practice remembering that just as there are two sides to us, there are two sides to all.

Are you seeing only the good in someone or can you see their shadow side as well?

compassion born from
true love is unattached to motive

Day 28
It's All Okay

Scrambling for security only ever brings temporary respite.

We are from generations and generations who have created opposites to a left or right, steering to a yes or no.

Think about how we change leg positions in meditation. Our legs hurt from sitting cross-legged, so we move them. Then we think, *Phew. What a relief!* Two minutes later, we want to move them again. We keep moving around seeking pleasure, seeking comfort; the satisfaction that we get is short-lived.

What if there were no right and wrong and everything simply is… if everything as it is is in its truthful and glorious presence?

coherence and existence is present now

Day 29
Neediness

Consider this: all day long we cling to our desire to repeat pleasant experiences, moving away from what is unpleasant. Despite all our efforts to remain in the pleasant we oscillate all day between the two.

Buddha's First Noble Truth is the existence of dukkha—a feeling of dissatisfaction that accompanies every experience in which we are identified with our needs.

The Buddha taught that it was the denial of this truth that is the cause of all suffering.

suffering comes from
pushing away the truth

Day 30
Three Aspects of Disappointment

Disappointment is usually comprised of three aspects:

The first is the anticipation of disappointment born from a memory of our past. This happens when we imagine some situation which might happen although it has not. We experience the disappointment as though it had already occurred.

The second is a moment when the disappointment happens, and we must somehow live through it. Usually we repeat our automatic default network response.

The third is living with the after-effects of lingering disappointment which are the stories we attach to our feelings.

we create space with daily practice;
we react in new healthy ways;
we suffer less

Day 31
No Worries

We have the power to create the future by forgiving and letting go of those stories of the past we allowed to define us. Knowing this, decide to let go of the painful experiences that cannot change. Commit to change what you can to make life more pleasant. List your greatest pains now.

fear is what has already happened;
what you do with the past in the present
effects your future

Day 32
Caring for Anxiety

A certain amount of nervousness in the external world is appropriate, yes. If we're not careful, we may drive off the road or, if someone is threatening us, we need to be alert.

Being in a state of fear all the time, however, is like locking oneself away from all beauty. The fear perpetuates until it is a way of life.

Learning to lay down the mistrust and embrace some uncertainty is a worthwhile lesson.

What conditions can you create where you can be honest and speak only truths? In what conditions do you feel love?

we are capable of adjusting
the volume of our trepidation

Day 33
Golden Questions

What do you do to avoid conflict, necessary though it may be?

What are you inclined to lie about, assuming that the truth might be intolerable?

What do you fake?

How does this serve you? Is there a deeper truth waiting behind the inauthentic?

to interview the self is to grow

Day 34
Honesty Is Peace

Yamas rest upon each other, as building blocks. Honesty follows ahimsa, nonviolence. In telling the truth we can take our time to express our words in harmony with ahimsa and an attitude of kindness.

Practicing satya and ahimsa together expands awareness of the effects your words and thoughts have on others and yourself.

Can you notice honesty is also a restraint through remaining silent if your words or thoughts are harmful?

knowing the effect our words have
on ourselves and others,
we can cause less harm

Day 35
Messages Gifted to Us

One great gift I received through teaching yoga was this note containing these words:

It's not about being able to do a pose; it's about the experience that people have when they come to your class.

Who is not aware they have inspired you?

What can you do for them?

Can you gift words of appreciation to someone today?

what we say to others is
a reflection of who we are

Day 36
The Joyful Narrative

We can choose not to listen to the voices that tell us to judge others, fear others, or harm others. Nor do we need to take responsibility for them. Others may be where we come from, but they aren't where we're going.

There is another voice, a voice of light that shines.

Ahimsa is a practice of listening to voices of lightness, creating a voice of light, believing the voice of light, then acting—based on that voice of light.

Notice today thoughts containing judgement, fear, or harm. Can you shine the voice of light that lives within you on them instead?

This is the practice of ahimsa, nonharming, nonviolent, in thoughts and actions.

we get to choose
the messages we listen to

Niyama: The 2nd Limb

"Yoga practice, both on and off the mat, opens up the heart by revealing our patterns of grasping and inflexibility. This practice leaves no stone unturned. Through a disciplined and appropriately designed yoga practice, we not only see clearly our conditioned ways of living, but we learn how to let go of those patterns so that our questions radically outnumber our answers. When we are open, and our habitual psychological and physical ways of being are suspended, we arrive in the present moments of life free to respond with an open and creative heart."
MICHAEL STONE, THE INNER TRADITION OF YOGA: A GUIDE TO YOGA PHILOSOPHY FOR THE CONTEMPORARY PRACTITIONER

The second branch, or limb, of Patañjali's yoga framework is niyama.

Niyama means rule, or laws. They are suggestions Patañjali provides as to inner awareness and observance which help us relate to ourselves.

Five smaller branches extend from the niyama, which Patañjali believes create a healthy inner environment, and establish self discipline, enabling you to live your highest quality life.

They are actions to practice to form patterns of growth:

1. Sauca: purity, cleanliness of mind, speech, and body. Sauca is two dimensional and both are interconnected:
    a. Outer cleanliness: the morning shower, washing hands after a bathroom visit.

b. Inner cleanliness: this includes purity of the mind. From drinking clean water to hydrate organs, to eliminating thoughts and emotions such as hate, anger, greed, and lust.

2. Santosa is contentment, acceptance, optimism. It is learning acceptance and peace, discovering joy, and being content—even when things are difficult. It includes accepting what you have, and being welcoming to yourself, and extending that to others. Active gratitude practice—routinely listing that for which you are thankful— is an excellent way to cultivate Santosa.

3. Tapas is persistence, perseverance, austerity. It's disciplined effort, focussing on goals. A way to incorporate tapas is to use creativity to assist with things you want to be disciplined about—for saving money it might mean leaving a credit card at home.

4. Svādhyāya is self-study, self-reflection, an intentional focus upon the self. This is done in asana, on the mat, and is a practice off the mat too. It is represented by the way you talk to yourself, the food you choose, and the quality and length of sleep you get. All these things affect the way you will feel the next day.

5. Īśvarapraṇidhāna is the contemplation of the divine. It involves surrendering to the divine. In practice, it is making choices that are for the good of all you are involved with.

The Niyama Days

Day 37
Nirvana

Suffering is caused by desire, the pursuit of pleasure, and material goods—all things that can never be satisfied. These have stories created around an "I," "me," or "mine." Acquiring material things and chasing cravings prolongs our suffering and adds to feelings of lack.

Nirvana is the freedom to extinguish these self-references. Achieving a state beyond—those worldly cycles of opposites our mind creates.

Can you observe these mind-wandering patterns when they arise, and can you let them pass through you?

nirvana is a state of being

Day 38
Eightfold Beauty

Buddha taught that following the Eightfold Path is the way to reach the state of nirvana. On this path are the eight practices: right view, right resolve, right speech, right conduct, right livelihood, right effort, right mindfulness, and right samadhi (meditative absorption or union). Which one will you practice today?

every moment is a stepping stone
on the energetic path to nirvana

Day 39
Glorious Vessel

Whole health depends on the reverence we have for the body that carries our wholeness around.

When we carry shame or guilt it is usually related to a childhood experience.

Releasing old stories allows us to shine brighter. In this way, letting go of shame, resentments, or experiences is letting glory and love thrive.

our bodies are vessels of
divine-loving potential

Day 40
Breath as a Bridge

When stress overwhelms the nervous system, the body is flooded with chemicals that prepare us for fight or flight.

It's a stress response that kicks in when we have to act quickly. When frequently activated by the stresses of everyday life, the stress chemicals can wear down a body and damage emotional health. Our breath is a bridge between our physical and spiritual worlds. Our breath is always there… like a best friend.

Guiding our attention to the breath throughout the day leaves a space between fight or flight where we can creatively respond. We can build our health and wellness.

Where do you feel your breath easily? At the nostrils or in the belly, rising and falling? Return to your breath as often as you can.

we can learn to respond
creatively to all situations

Day 41
Power of Myth

It is unrealistic to think one person completes us… that there is a perfect match—our other half—who will fit together with us in all ways and with whom we can share every aspect of our lives.

Such ideas are based on the ancient Greek myth, told by Plato, that we were each a whole split into two… and somewhere, out there, our other true half was waiting… or searching for us and when we reunite we would find true love.

This myth became the foundation for Western romanticism; its foundation is not rooted in reality. To believe in it is like believing in the handsome prince astride a white horse who sweeps up the fair, incomplete maiden.

We now have consciousness to accept a new story. I am whole. No one is coming for me. I am. I am the one I have been waiting for.

we are whole—all we seek is within

Day 42
Your Hero's Journey

Yoga is a spiritual path that leads inwards, towards your heart.

It is a hero's journey during which you will traverse valleys of darkness and meet a cast of characters including: anxiety, sadness, anger, pride, jealousy.

Along the way you will have many opportunities to develop the tool of an equanimous mind—calm and composed—so you can be strong, brave, courageous, resilient, confident, optimistic, responsible, and compassionate.

Which of your greatest characteristics did you learn from darkness?

life is a training ground; yoga is
a masterclass for navigating the journey

Day 43
Not Knowing Is Home

Realize: all of your ideas of knowing block you from the truth—more than they serve to reveal it. It has been shared from sages that it is when you think you know something that you are actually lost.

not knowing is intimacy,
the best path home

Day 44
Noticing Patterns

The first step to eradicating negative thoughts is to discover them. Self-doubt or lack of confidence manifest out of patterns of negative thinking.

Do you have a stream of thoughts that pop up daily and make you doubt your self-worth? When you notice patterns, you can work with them or let them go.

The mind is a garden. Tend to each thought as if planting a seed. If we are not tending to our thoughts the weeds grow. If we nurture good thoughts, we create positive patterns.

when we identify, explore, express
gratitude, we allow flow

Day 45
Compassionate Living

The challenging times are often made challenging—by us.

People don't do things to us, they just do things.

If someone wounds your heart, instead of understanding or reasoning or searching for the weapon, turn your attention, as a mother cares for her baby, to care for the hole in your own heart.

caring for your heart
is caring for the universe

Day 46
Chalice of Honour

Imagine making such a distinction in your own life to honor the things and people you love with a brand of caring expressed in a manner of appreciation that only their loss can provide.

In yoga class, in your romantic relationships, as a parent, and in your work, you are gathering your attention into little cups of intention, values, and effort. It is wonderful that human beings have this capacity.

To attain freedom in your life, drink from each of those cups as though they were broken.

honour from a sacred place
of imagined absence

Day 47
Hello Me

Who do you spend the most time with? Your spouse? Your best friend? Your children? Your co-workers?

You spend the most time with yourself, which is why the tone and content of your internal dialogue is incredibly important to how you feel about yourself.

You have to be completely okay with being alone.

we are completely and thoroughly
immersed in our own company

Day 48
Managing Process

Being a yogi, reiki master, and meditation teacher means I am open, raw, and vulnerable most days. I struggle with feeling the suffering of others. I grapple with the gap between how I see things are as opposed to how I believe things should be, based on my own lessons from my life experiences. Meditation closes this gap.

I'm guilty of holding onto strong beliefs and feelings. I am not proud to have acted from them. I forgive myself. I remind myself that I am enough. I am abundant. I sail on waves of the sea. I can go with the flow. The universe provides for my needs. I am thankful for what I have.

What are these processes like for you?

there is nowhere to "get to"
we are already here

Day 49
Give Infinitely

We want to feel in the right.

We want it to be recognized that someone, something, has done us wrong.

If possible, we want an admission of guilt.

In looking for this type of moral closure, we give away our power. We're saying, "I cannot move past this experience until…"

Opposites are mental bars keeping us from intimacy and self-love. What we truly require is an internal, emotional shift. The outside world cannot take care of our feelings.

What do you need to hear to feel better? Write to yourself everything you wish to hear.

we can apologize, acknowledge,
hug, or gift ourselves any of these
in any moment

Day 50
Valued Roles

Embrace being the caretaker of your garden. Take pride in the tools you use to root out that which is not wanted. Take time in learning about all the varieties of plants that will thrive. Enrich the soil in which everything grows.

What nourishes you?

your garden is sacred

Day 51
Magnificence

As you cultivate and become awestruck at the seedlings of love, kindness, and compassion that sprout, marvel at the peaceful buds that develop. Enjoy the garden of your mind, slow and truly stop and smell the roses.

the balance of nature exists in you

Day 52
Clarity

It is easy to blame another or avoid an issue. Taking the full responsibility on our own shoulders is difficult.

Humility comes into play when we can look at ourselves in the mirror and admit we are at fault, at least partly at fault.

We can learn to ask: What is my role in the drama? We can look for the root as we would in gardening. The stronger our skill of finding and pulling roots, the freer our mind. We are here to break ancestral patterns and create new pathways for the future.

there can be great relief and release in recognizing our role

Day 53
Heart Truth

Pushing to get what we want through sideways accusation or complaint is normal for many. We tend not to straight-out say what we long for because it exposes our vulnerability.

Can you go into the discomfort, then speak the truth of your heart knowing you are interconnected and every word matters… that you matter?

vulnerability is magnificently brave

Day 54
Vocal Lessons

Emotions are like a compass; they alert us to which direction we go, they light the path. Emotions are our natural intelligence. Let them guide. Apologize for actions not feelings.

For some, when they are driven by feeling, they often feel shame about what is seen as abnormal emotionality.

Can we break free of the shackles of shame and guilt which permeate our culture and impose silence on the soul?

Yes, we can share… yes, we must contribute our voices. Who are we if we don't rise to greet new awareness with courage?

we are meant to trust the heart's wisdom
and hear the heart's voice of love

Day 55
Cautious

We prefer to stay safely guarded behind our complaints. It is easier to focus on what our partner isn't giving us. If we never share what we want outright, they could never reject us. Right?

Wrong.

What we often get in response is distance. This feels like rejection.

Ironically, it is the very act of showing our heart in this naked way that has the power to create the deep intimacy we long for.

What skills do you need to bury the story of rejection? What words will guide you to share your heart and bring you closer to intimacy?

if we feel we're hiding something
or ourselves, then we probably are;
we can now share what is in our heart

Day 56
Love Actually

How do we assess the balance of love? How do we know if we are giving too much and not receiving enough in return?

The Dalai Lama says: "Selfless love is often misunderstood. It is not a question of neglecting oneself for others' benefit. In fact, when you benefit others, you benefit yourself because of the principle of interdependence. I want to stress the importance of enlarging your mind and bringing the sufferings of others onto yourself."

the capacity to give yourself and others
love and to receive love from yourself
and from others is infinite

Day 51
Reruns

Disappointment has a chimerical quality—fantastically visionary—because our minds refuse to accept what is. We relive the disappointment over and over, rarely noticing that after the initial experience it is only a memory, that we are re-experiencing, much like watching old movie reruns.

Are you playing horror movies in your mind?

Do you know it's the same mind that can create comedies and love stories? You are the one you have been waiting for. Flip any script that keeps you feeling and living in old, harmful, or destructive patterns.

What scares you now?

Can you create a love story of the situation/relationship?

you are nature; you are meant to grow
and, to grow, you have to let go;
you can transform fear into love

Day 58
Lessons in Patience

Occasions and situations which require patience are also opportunities that gift us moments.

The best use of each moment is to take notice of the blessings in our life and say thank you.

Often, we become fixated on what we don't have. This focus becomes an obsession which can create a negative spiral in all areas of life—making the wait more difficult.

By turning our focus on what we already have, and are grateful for, we begin to attract people, things, and situations that are positive and healthy.

What are you grateful for in this moment?

When we are in gratitude, we are a magnetic force.

Create conditions in your life to make gratitude lists, gratitude jars, gratitude journals.

gratitude is a natural healing modality

Day 59
Loving Speech

Your words have energy. They can help or hurt. Ask yourself before speaking: Is it kind? It is helpful? Does it improve on silence?

Silence, and not communicating, eventually turns against you. Speak your truth when opportunities present themselves.

Face the chaos of your making. Move forward honourably. Show others who you are. Share yourself as a voice of clarity.

your essence includes your voice

Day 60
Mirror

I am here.

Self-care became lost. How can we give to others if we are broken?

Self-care is an essential caregiving act.

Sadly, we cannot help others by actions that attempt to "help" or "fix" them, but we can model self-care so fiercely until we become a mirror and example for others to care for themselves.

when we shine our brightest,
we give others permission to shine as well

Day 61
Know Thyself

Banish the superficial and move beyond the inconsequential.

A true healer is the one who heals themself first so others can benefit from their own healing.

Who are you?

What do you stand for?

walk your path, take your stand,
be your best carer

Day 62
Healing Trajectory

Meaning rectifies the tragedies of life.

Aim toward what you choose. You are moving anyway so why not point your sail in the direction you want to go? If you decide it's not a fit, you can always change course.

flow love in the direction
your heart whispers

Asana: The 3rd Limb

"If you perform asanas regularly, you will feel more flexible physically and emotionally. Flexibility is the essential difference between the vitality of youth and the lassitude of old age. Here is a yogic expression that we find inspiring: 'Infinite flexibility is the secret to immortality.'"

DEEPAK CHOPRA, *The Seven Spiritual Laws of Yoga:
A Practical Guide to Healing Body, Mind, and Spirit*

Asana is position. The most well-known limb of the eightfold path of yoga, it often gets interpreted as yoga itself. When we say we are going to do a yoga class, we mean we're going to do an asana class.

Asana means comfortable seat. Earlier asanas were exactly as the position describes: seated positions readying us for meditation. In seated meditation monks would stretch their legs into these poses so they could sit in stillness without ache for longer periods.

Physical work is necessary to achieve union of our energy systems—called wholeness. This is where asana comes in: poses are a way to quiet the mind. A healthy body—without pain—is an ideal environment for concentration, meditation, and joyful connection.

The body cannot live without the mind. Negative thoughts are as unhealthy as physical stress. There is an optimum state for the body and mind to thrive.

Patañjali teaches that asana keeps the body steady for meditation, and meditation prepares us to master thought patterns which, in turn, leads us to self-realization.

As you encounter challenging poses, focus on your feelings: are you breathing?

If you cannot hold the pose, ease up and be gentle with your progress. Let yourself grow into the challenges. Don't force, just feel.

The goal is unification of the mental and physical energies. Asana helps each practitioner experience this bliss of alignment.

The body is always present, even when the mind is wandering. That is why coming back to the body is a great tool for helping silence the mind. The body strives for balance, homeostasis, and wholeness. Asana practice creates conditions for such love, kindness, and compassion.

The Asana Days

Day 63
Heart of Asana

An open heart loves the world. It sings to the sun and tells stories to the moon. Yoga supports our hero's journey to the infinite ocean of being.

there is so much power within our heart

Day 64
Deep Roots

As a beginner, standing poses are your starting point for growth and stability. As a more seasoned practitioner, practicing standing poses maintains that strength and stability.

when our feet are firmly planted
into the earth, the winds of change
may bend us; we will not break

Day 65
Sageness

Yoga can support the whole being if the student is open to the process.

How open a student is often depends on how teachers embody the lessons and display their own understanding. Heart centred teachers who fully embody a yogic lifestyle demonstrate an essence and energy in their teachings.

As a teacher, how do you portray your heart in practice, in life? Can you hear your heart's voice?

we are all expanding our mastery

Day 66
Wheels of Energy

Chakrasana comes from the word chakra, which means wheel in Sanskrit—since the posture resembles a wheel.

It is a deep back bend demanding flexibility and strength—and it requires it at the same time from different parts of the body including the shoulders, arms, wrists, abdominals, back, legs, and glutes. It is one of the most effective ways to open the front of the body.

Notice how your back bends today. Bask in the glory of your spine's natural curves and abilities. Embrace how the circle symbolizes continuous energy, flow, and continuity.

we are all expanding and
coming home to ourselves

Day 67
Breathe

The pigeon pose stretches the thighs, groins, and abdomen. It can often be felt deeply in specific upper-leg and hip muscles, including the psoas, piriformis, TFL (tensor fascia latae), and gluteus maximus. It relieves tension in the chest and shoulders and stimulates the abdominal organs that help to regulate digestion.

Can you be brave enough to make modifications to support your practice? Can you fall in love with this deep stretch? If you lose the feeling of your breath, you've gone too far. Find a balance between effort and ease.

the value of being in posture
is to connect with our breath

Day 68
Perception

Reverse warrior is a demanding posture. Within all the moving parts are a lot of alignment issues on which to focus.

When practiced mindfully, this posture can be amazing for the body.

Do you love this pose? Dislike this pose?

The mind will create opposites of your liking or disliking the pose, stopping you at form. Can you feel beyond any storytelling?

let feelings and sensations flow, there is more—yoga is never what you think; it's always revolutionizing

Day 69
Practice of Remembering

Let your body be your teacher.

You spend most of your day in your head. A yoga class is a good time to draw attention inside the body and outside the mind. To achieve this, we use an object for our attention to return to. The breath is such an object. Bring your attention to your breath as often as you can. This will develop focus, awareness, and concentration.

The tendency of the mind is to wander. That's okay. Come back to your breath over and over again. Each breath is a new opportunity. The breath is always inside, like a best friend.

your breath is a
homecoming to the present

Day 70
Heart Opener

The camel pose, or ustrasana, brings something unique to asana practice. It is a heart-opening posture with the chest toward the sky. As you breathe here, what can you open up to? What has to be let go for a shift to occur? Can you allow the answers to flow without attaching stories?

Be brave, knowing you are safe and the universal laws highlight that the best is always yet to come. Letting go is also self-love.

Visualize your chest full of rays of sunshine. Pour golden light through your body—from head to toes. Do you need to write something on paper? Can you then transform it into a love story?

we are the creator of our universe
and master of our experiences

Day 71
Good Vibrations

Backbends are an incredible challenge, creating a vulnerability of self… this is often something we avoid (being vulnerable).

If we think of the camel pose as a part of our own journey, our courageous openness will be rewarded with a unique destination. The reward is always a more pleasant state of being.

we dwell in possibilities,
abundance, fullness, and more
than we could ever imagine

Day 72
Love the Pause

There is a natural pause at the very end of the exhale; the inhale springs up from that pause. Can you feel it? You can practice enjoying that pause. You can enjoy the pause like you enjoy sunshine. This pause is a gift of freedom from thought. A mind free from disturbances is… yoga.

we dwell in grace, possibility,
and abundance—everything is
happening for us

Day 73
In the Middle

Stillness is cultivated by practice and using an object for meditation, such as the breath. Stillness quiets the chatter of the mind and we notice we are more than our thoughts. There is space between our thoughts and our reactions. We experience our loving interconnected nature beyond storytelling. This state is beyond the five senses, a wellspring of knowledge, peace, and love. Have you noticed you never quite get where you're going and something is always arising for you to handle?

We are always in the middle.

With every practice, your heart softens.

Let your cup overflow.

Practice until your world changes.

Create new beliefs through this power of yoga.

our home is our heart—the heartbeat of
the world is the same heart beating in
your chest right now

Day 74
Stand Your Ground

Standing poses are an essential element of asana for those whose bodies allow. When standing, practice feeling equal weight between your front and back foot. You can play by leaning back onto the back foot and then to the front. See if you can find a spot in the middle. Imagine every exhale confirming your connection to the earth… each inhale drawing earth's energy up into your body.

When we feel strong in yoga class, our body will remember off the mat. We create, through our physical practice, new pathways of strength. From that, all good things will begin to emerge in our life. Strength is required to align our lifestyle and relationships with the wisdom of our heart.

the strength of the earth is within us,
connecting us to our
highest potential for growth

Day 15
Embodied Self-Love

We cultivate self-love with intense self-trust, wisdom, and discernment; attunement to physical signals; and deep connection with intuition.

Old patterns quiet down with our new self-appreciation and supportive actions. Trust and bathe in your glory as you grow through this process. You are creating the greatest love you have ever dreamed of: you.

we practice yoga not to become enlightened, we practice because we remember we already are

Day 76
Mantra

Mantra means sacred message in Sanskrit. Positive energy vibrations regulate our chemical imbalances, calm the nervous system, and create an overall sense of wellbeing.

Mantras enhance states of relaxation by engaging positive brainwaves including alpha, gamma, delta.

Chanting (repeating a mantra) helps quiet mental noise by reeling in your scattered thoughts and focussing on a single word or phrase.

Mantra practice can be used to deal with struggles, challenges, or conflicts. A calming mantra is: I am peaceful, or I matter.

mantras allow us to
experience more pleasantness

Day 77
Nurture the Sacred

Like a gardener who envisions the seed they planted bursting into a blossoming perennial, so can a mantra be thought of as a seed for energizing an intention. Much in the same way we plant a flower seed, we plant mantras in the fertile soil of practice. Post them up on your mirrors, computer, fridge, or any frequently seen space as reminders. Nurtured, over time, the mantra will produce and bear the fruit of your intention.

yogis are great gardeners

Day 78
Mantra Magic

The mind wanders. Just as we use breath as an object to create space for our nature to arise, reciting a mantra will plant positive self-talk seeds into your mind boosting your strength and power.

Think of mantras as being postures for your mind, the way asanas are physical postures. They are often used like affirmations to stay connected to a particular state of mind. Mantras like, "I am strong," "I am focused," or "I let go and surrender," can help the practitioner maintain a connection to the state they wish to cultivate during their time on the mat.

meaningful sacred words invoke a
vibrational frequency which resonates
throughout the universe

Day 79
Hand in Hand

Vipassana meditation works well with hatha yoga because the latter helps with grounding in the current moment through body awareness. This helps the meditation experience. Conversely, the mindful practice supports new thoughts and feelings about the hatha practice.

collaboration harmonizes

Day 80
Comprehension

When we practice hatha and vipassana what follows is a greater clarity of thought and action.

Vipassana is an insight practice. Once our stillness becomes a container for thought to roam freely—like clouds in the sky—vippasana enters insight. At that point, you will hear your heart speaking to you.

When we begin to learn how the mind works, we can control it and not have it control us. We can create conditions to use it to our advantage.

thinking is of the mind; it is your heart
that has a wisdom that is boundless
and pure potential

Day 81
Do The Work

When we deal with a physical injury within ourselves, we can approach our yoga teacher with a goal of "fix this injury, please" in the way that there will be relief from the discomfort and the limitation the injury brings with it.

It is better to bring mindfulness to the injury, otherwise the pain may be relieved in the short term, based on a quick fix. Later it can become chronic pain or a more serious injury.

Examine the disturbance in the body's natural balance by reviewing what conditions have come together.

wellness has space to grow when the root of
what is no longer serving you is discovered

Day 82
Healing

Discomfort is a signal of imbalance. There is no reason to organize around it. Instead, use discomfort as a navigational tool... to track the origin and to record your path of healing—when the discomfort eases, that is the indication you are on a healing path.

With the help of a yoga teacher, and perhaps a wise medical professional, use questions to uncover underlying conditions, including how you hold and move the body, your emotional life, and your beliefs concerning your body. Self-inquiry and stillness can provide the answers. No stillness=no insight.

What do you believe about your body?

you have all you need to heal yourself

Day 83
On Track

A mantra is a great tool to bring awareness to what is happening in the here and now. Mantra-induced awareness disturbs the narrative of the wandering mind. Mantras help you by training attention so you stay with your present experience.

Mantras are also selected to create intention for a day, a month, a season, or longer. Be adventuresome with your practice. Have fun. Always learn.

practice your mantra today
as a tool for life

Day 84
Seedling

Trust the process. Everything is constantly changing. Everything is impermanent. Use this trust to form new attitudes and ways of living.

You'll be tested for everything you want; the universe presents lots of practice opportunities.

Walk the path of your heart, and you will meet masters who will offer their guidance and wisdom.

Each milestone we pass, a new one appears. Each time we leave a piece of ourselves behind as sentient seedlings, we also grow. We are ever evolving.

What do you want to leave in this world to make it a better place for future generations?

growth is inevitable—now is the time to
create the life you want

Day 85
Lean Into You

Find length in your side body, from the back of your heel, rooted to your fingertips, with extended side angle pose.

Sometimes there are problems with this pose... keeping the back heel anchored to the floor when bending the knee, and not being able to touch the fingertips of the lower hand to the floor.

A solution for the first issue is to brace your back heel against the wall then, as you bend the knee and lower your torso to the side, visualize your heel pushing the wall away.

On the second problem: settle your forearm on top of the bent knee rather than bringing it down to the floor. Or use a block outside the front foot to support the hand.

when you modify a yoga posture, you are making a good decision for yourself

Day 86
Comfort

The lotus pose, known as padmasana, is believed to be the best position for long sessions of seated meditation. Because if a meditating person fell asleep in lotus pose, they would not fall over.

While the lotus pose is grounding and awesome for stabilization, a person does not have to do lotus pose to meditate or practice yoga.

Lotus is a pose that demands a lot from the joints. It's not for everyone. And that's okay.

Create your own meditation pose today or your own version of lotus.

you are more than your thoughts

Day 87
Purposed Passion

Yoga lifestyle welcomes us to set intentions for our life and for our practice. It supports us with skills to create conditions to live the intentions and builds up our strength, bravery, and courage through asana and mental practices.

our intentions are living, breathing things

Day 88
Every Part Is Essential

Yoga is attuned to the body on the basic dimensions of physical, body, mind, and emotions. Yoga guides us to the heart and shows us, through practice, how to love all the bits and pieces that scare us into looking away. Yoga is a path of the self, through the self, to the self. It exposes the greatness within you.

every cell is pure, loving energy

Day 89
Sharing

As you experience the powerful alignment between body, mind, soul, and energy, your self-realization and self-love will increase. It is essential to care for the body the best ways you can.

Who are you not to share your gifts or shine brightly on, for, and in this world? Rise into the power of being. Realize the immortality of human nature.

your body is your vessel
to experience life

Day 90
Intimacy

Yoga teaches self-care, self-appreciation, and self-love. The practice introduces each of us to our innermost self, the absolute core of our being.

We become most intimate with our capacity to simply be, also known as our Buddha nature.

we are like water—ever-changing, perfectly imperfect potential

Day 91
Deeper Bonds

Hatha yoga describes the action of one body part holding another as binding, or when two body parts are intertwined. When practiced properly, binding allows the body to relax and go deeper into a pose, as well as promoting a longer held pose.

A bind is a way to express creativity, to play with a pose and be your own leader.

Can you find a bind to try today?

hold on slowly, steadily, deeply

Day 92
Discovery

If you practice, you will find:

- Your mind is cooler, clearer, and less biased
- A deeper connection to the present moment
- An awareness that your emotions are not reality

All these discoveries will affect how you interpret experiences… which can lead to interacting with the world more easily as well as improved relationships and kindness towards yourself.

practice makes perfect clarity

Day 93
The Little Engine of You

If you're new to yoga or meditation and you don't think you can do it, chances are you won't. The execution of an asana starts to happen in the mind, then it manifests into your body. If a yoga pose looks difficult, work first on believing you can do it.

I think I can, I think I can

Day 94
Invisible Protector

Truth is, you just don't know where you'll end up. You don't know what situations will arise. The body keeps the score for you as you move through the poses and of each minute of practice.

Trust the yoga. Yoga practice is important because it keeps a safe foundation within. A foundation free of stimulants and toxins, free of negativity, and free of fear.

Yoga is a much-needed bodyguard, an energy guard, and a mind guard that we need because of the world we're living in today—technology and instant gratification at the touch of our fingers.

self-love, self-compassion,
and understanding is a superpower
and protective shield

Day 95
Foundational

A yoga foundation within is built like the foundation of a home. One piece of practice at a time. One tool or technique at a time. One yoga class at a time. One breath at a time.

Major restoration projects of this kind take courage and dedication, loyalty, and responsibility.

These values and morals accumulate. They are powers within each of us. You can do this. I can do this. We can do this. They can do this. Everyone can build a foundation within themselves, to stand strong and steady no matter what situations arise.

Your life is happening for you, not to you. Can you feel it?

all life happens for me

Day 96
Mountain Stream Clear

What is required of us is that we are prepared for every eventuality—that we learn to live happily with impermanence and change. Keep this in mind as you flow through poses today.

Where do you get stuck?

What can you offer yourself to move freely?

water washes away mud,
yoga cleanses too

Day 97
Healer Warrior

It takes great courage to become unstuck. When we free ourselves, we change the way we perceive reality. Though the outcome of the change is magnificent, the changing part can feel chaotic. We are unravelling the sweater that we have worn for a lifetime. Then we are knitting it into a robe.

As you practice, take note of the chaos and breathe through it; take note of the new results and breathe them in. Watch the rows unravel, watch the ball of wool grow, and watch yourself create the new garment.

everything flows, everything changes.
Yoga is a catalyst to change—the fruit
being self-love, the balm that soothes the
wounds inside

Day 98
Understanding

Sometimes things don't work out. It can happen that you arrive at yoga class desperate for calm and there are disruptive students or a teacher is distracted. Other times your racing mind overpowers the relaxation you expected to get from the warm-up or sun salutations.

Suddenly there's a pain or discomfort and your hopes are dashed—or it seems that way. You begin to beat yourself up: why am I always injured? How come I don't keep up my practice at home? And it's not just in yoga class. It may seem in your whole life you can not do anything right. When you notice this natural tendency: Stop. Breathe. Love. Respond. Intend.

there is always so much more

Day 99
Balancing

In becoming an adult, you learned how to cope with disappointment—otherwise you wouldn't be able to function at all. Yet, the conundrum remains: if you've learned to live with disappointments, then why does it still take so much of your energy to cope with them?

Why do you get sad, depressed, worried, irritated, moody, anxious, grumpy, lethargic, or nonresponsive, not just occasionally, perhaps many times over a day or a week—sometimes in small ways, sometimes big?

Where is the yoga in all this reactivity?

Yoga expands our capacity for positive emotions, less reactivity, and ultimately less suffering of these strong emotions.

question your feelings, interview you,
add some yoga bliss as needed

Day 100
Unnecessary Identification

Hatha yoga offers an opportunity to be free of identification.

Note how sometimes you observe your mind wanting your body to be able to do something, and then notice how you identify with that desire—the level of frustration and disappointment when the body can't do it.

None of that desire helps you do yoga.

What skill or technique can you offer yourself to create a more loving yoga practice for you?

freedom is clarity

Day 101
River of Life

When you choose life as a teacher, life never disappoints… it only offers itself for practice. Being with life is to practice yoga.

When disappointment occurs, the practice is to realize, *I'm lost in disappointment. I've confused myself with a desire, therefore identified with it, which is now causing me to suffer.*

It is not that the physical or emotional pain that accompanies disappointment is unreal; of course pain hurts. But it passes.

Perhaps you can view yourself as an explorer making your life an adventure.

be with life

Day 102
Love Is All

Shine a light on your disappointments. Hold a blanket around your sadness. Offer a shoulder to your suffering. Bring a tea to your sorrow. If you can guide yourself through all of life, then you will be truly aligned with life.

there is a compass, a compassion,
within each of us

Day 103
Sculpt and Mold

By practicing positive thought patterns (affirmations) repetitively, we create new connections in the areas of the brain that process what we are thinking about.

Your spoken and intentional positive affirmations prove you are special, you are enough, you are intelligent, you are worthy of love, you are valuable.

Remember and/or create an affirmation now. You can do great things.

affirmations are tools of cultivation

Day 104
Reduction

Minimalists give up excess belongings that cause stress and distraction. Decluttering follows the same path: it obliges you to go through your belongings so that you only retain—hence, own—what sparks joyfulness… what you can happily manage. Clearing clutter creates space on the outside and the inside.

What can you do with new space?

less is often more

Day 105
Outcome

What is the goal of asana practice?

The pursuit of quieting the mind and truly listening to the body, right?

Notice how you feel about your body after your practice. Capture this feeling, carry it around with you, and share it with those nearby.

sharing is caring

Day 106
Again

Repeating a meditational pose is beneficial; it impacts the formation of a faithful practice. In effect, the seat becomes one of truth—our own truth. Daily meditation practice is a commitment to ourselves.

there is great beauty in ritual

Day 107
Absolution

I forgive myself for my mistakes. We all make mistakes. I used to feel regret about some of my mistakes because I am a good person and want to do the best I can.

Now, I am still a good person, and I release all feelings of regret because I have learned a lesson and moved on.

I forgive myself for errors I have made—I have felt badly about them long enough. I have suffered enough, and now it is time to be free. By freeing myself from past mistakes, I can move on and do kinder things. I forgive myself.

life is abundant;
we are destined for breakthroughs
and we can free our own mind

Day 108
Circle Creating

Choose people who want things to be better. Choose people who strive towards dreams. It's a good thing, not a selfish thing, to choose people who are good for you. Be around those who are happy when they see your life get better and be a person who is happy to see the lives of others improve. List a positive, passionate human you can count on now, so this, too, begins your circle of trust.

we decide who we spend time with

Day 109
Be Bold

Be your own sun. Shine on yourself. Shine on others. Be your own song. Sing to yourself. Sing out loud.

Be your own door. Carry yourself over your own threshold. Invite people in. Dearest one, you can and these are acts aligned with dwelling in possibility.

What does an openness of endless possibilities feel like in your body?

boldly experience the now

Day 110
I See

There is a crucial difference between past and future. The past is fixed and can only recycle memory. The future can become your wildest dream or simply be made better. Your past is linked to conditioned reactions, the future is available for you to create.

A vision board is a great tool to visualize what you'd like to create for the future. Explore magazines and cut out images, words, or quotes which resonate with you in your future. Before sleep is a great time for this. Paste those images or words into a collage of your future. Display your board where you can see it every day.

look through the window of now

Day III
Enjoy the View

When you're walking up the hill, look to the sides of the road, take your shoes off, and wander into the grassy verges. When you are climbing that mountain, take breaks by sitting on felled trees and their stumps.

In yoga, enjoy the way to the pose, take your time along the route… slowly bring yourself there.

the climb offers magnificent vistas

Day 112
Moving Target

An aim is like an intention. Having an aim means you have something in your sights. Having something in your sights means a purpose has been identified. Purpose and passion are the best of friends. Be passionate. Be purposeful.

Could you apply an aim in each pose? Can you then apply this aim in your life?

loving intention sets our sails
to the direction we want to reach

Day 113
Bye Dragon

To that voice in my head that still wonders if I'm good enough, if anyone likes me, if I've got what it takes, and that casts a lingering shadow of doubt over everything—you are a paper dragon, it is with gratitude I let you rest in peace now.

I choose faith. Now kindly step aside so I can get back to work.

Practice your poses with this new energy.

shake it up, set it free,
and rise from the ashes

Day 114
Beautiful Bounty

One of the most rewarding spiritual practices is to cultivate the ability to bring love into all aspects of your life and to all people you encounter.

How can you cultivate a loving presence today?

Today, when you see another person, say silently: the light in me salutes the light in you.

we are intricately and essentially
interconnected by seeds of love; plant many

Day 115
Sugar and Spice

Practice poses tailored to your needs. Look to experienced instructors to guide you, and concentrate on proper alignment to avoid serious injury.

You are unique, that includes every cell in your body. Poses are significant. Your physical body must be a priority. If you feel any ripping or pulling sensations, you've gone too far. Can you add sweetness by releasing your jaw and softly smiling?

Where is the balance between effort and ease in each pose for you?

awareness and willingness
are keys to progress

Day 116
Heartache Help Aid

There have been times when tears have streamed down my face in savasana and I was eternally grateful that the room was dark.

More than that, I was grateful to have had the loving support of like-minded community members, where I felt comfortable enough to go to class during times of sorrow—because it helped me move through my daily life after I'd moved and strengthened my body on my mat.

My teacher taught me: "You do some of your best work with a broken heart."

Sadness offers sensitivity to a wide range of feelings.

what we do with our darkness
will help us shine

Day 117
Grace

Growth is natural. Rivers change courses. Saplings appear from seeds. Forests flourish, then burn and renew.

All things are impermanent. They arise, and they pass away.

To live in harmony with this truth brings much pleasantness.

Bring this into your movement practice; embody being pleasant as you move throughout your day.

you are the seed, you are the tree,
you are grace

Day 118
Gratitude

We can speak our thanks after something has happened, and that is wonderful. We can show our thanks after something has happened, and that is powerful. Beyond that, we can speak and show our thanks *before* something has happened, and that is profoundly foresighted and manifestational.

a grateful life is a proactive
and profound existence

Day 119
Calm Body

Yoga minimizes the physical effects of stress on the body. By encouraging relaxation, yoga will help lower the levels of the stress hormones, like cortisol, in your body.

What does yoga do for you?

de-stress over distress

Day 120
Dig with Kindness

The spiritual energy released during yoga class strips away all that is false. Most of us begin a spiritual practice having known only our false selves. As those layers begin to fall away, it can feel, at first, as if we are going backward instead of forward. Practice erodes the edifice we built of our false self.

Suddenly, our whole way of knowing, of doing, of being comes into question. Our certainties fall away, along with the persona we've long presented to the world. Many of us find we have built our houses on sand, and the lives we've created cannot stand up to the heat of our practice. We may lose a job, relationships, old friendships, and other things. We stand once more as a child in the world, open and empty.

Invite this process into your asana practice. Greet whatever arises with kindness. Kindness unsticks what has served its purpose. Kindness allows that which has served its purpose to flow away, creating spaciousness in your mind.

a kind attitude softens the release of what has served its purpose, creating space for all good things

Day 121
Ascension

Becoming aware of our choices, we move toward more loving decisions. We no longer limit our love.

It is a process to learn awareness and to master the art of conscious decisions. And that is okay. Being a student of life is an honor. Being alive is everything.

Where do you feel most alive?

we are the student, apprentice, and master

Day 122
Life Link

When we live every day in survival mode, we're attempting to force, control, and push outcomes. That is the way of the ego.

When we live in a state of conscious peace and trust, we never need to force how things will turn out or come to be. Because in that state we are filled with trust and we know we are connected to something greater. We end up being grateful for things before they have even happened because we feel like they have happened.

This is the way of peace for the body, mind, and soul. The journey to wholeness.

What can you be grateful for today?

the more loving our connections,
the greater our connection to the loving

Day 123
Write Life

How do you want to speak to yourself?

Exploring the answer to that question through writing, then reading what you have written, will set forth a whole new pathway in the brain. Write yourself a love story. The action of writing onto paper, is a powerful force.

Can you notice resistance before writing, and then write anyway?

all expression is simply a stream of consciousness... a river of intentional words

Day 124
Let It Pour

Intention for yoga practice today:
  Grace is like rain. Ego is an umbrella blocking grace and miracles. Embrace the mindset of *I am graceful on my mat today.*

splash in the puddles, dance in grace

Day 125
Everybody. Anybody. Somebody. Your Body

Be selective to whom you give your attention. People often want your presence or what you materially have. You must discern your value, your worth.

Many can tell a story to wield a specific result from you. Whilst meditatively listening, silently ask yourself: what is their role in the drama? Is there a secondary gain?

Go through your phone contacts and friend lists today, and routinely applying this wisdom.

a few true kindred spirits
are worth more than any large group

Pranayama: The 4th Limb

"Breathing in, I calm body and mind. Breathing out, I smile.
Dwelling in the present moment I know this is the only moment."
THICH NHAT HANH, *BEING PEACE*

Pranayama is the fourth limb of the eightfold path of yoga. Prana represents the life force and the energy that constantly flows through the bodies of all living creatures.

Pranayama is the act of moving energy by directing the breath. When we use breathing to support our intentions, the results are spectacular. More fresh air in the body means more oxygen to the organs. Using specific breathing techniques means more flexibility in situations whether they are challenging poses or stressful incidents. Breathing deeply signals our parasympathetic nervous system to calm the body, ease our fears, and reduce anxiety.

Practiced breathing techniques will create a balanced respiration even when not actively practicing. The body remembers each breathing practice and misses it when you don't practice. In a similar way to how you sense when you forgot to brush your teeth, you will become attuned in response to remembering your breath and or pranayama practice.

Turning attention to your breath in yoga class is a technique that anchors your attention and strengthens the act of remembering, as the mind wanders, coming back to your breath on a moment to moment basis is powerful. Since the body is in the present moment, feeling each inhale and exhale, allows us to feel fully present. Breath is a natural medicine, and pranayama is a skill.

When breath and pose are brought together, it's a purification for the body and mind.

Begin to observe your breath in different situations. Then, change your breath by lengthening an inhale, exhale, or both, and pay attention to subtle changes arising and passing. Have fun; every breath is fresh.

The Pranayama Days

Day 126
Breath

We get caught up in doing rather than being. We can find it difficult to picture complete calmness. Yet it is through quiet that we can hold joy in the palm of our hand and watch it dance. Through concentration on breathing we can dance with joy.

For this day, bring awareness to your breath as often as you can.

our breath is always there,
like our best friend

Day 127
Bridging

Many of us relax in front of our screened devices at the end of the day, essentially checking out of life and into chaos.

A better way to handle stress is to practice actual relaxation techniques, including a focus on breathing in and out, so that between the practices of yoga and meditation we can still feel them active within us.

No one can avoid stress. We can counteract detrimental effects from stress by learning how to engage in a flowing state. A relaxation response returns us to calm. Each time we become conscious of breath, we build a bridge. A bridge between one moment and the next, and between the world of our five senses and the ethereal one.

Close your eyes. Do you feel your breath at your nostrils or do you feel it in your belly rising and falling?

relaxation is essential;
breath connects the mental and physical

Day 128
Intake

The next time negative thoughts start to crop up, consciously pause what you are doing and observe. Notice how the thoughts make your body feel. What part of your body holds those feelings? Consciously feel these thoughts and, just as consciously, take a series of deep, cleansing breaths. Practice noticing the negatives as they arise; invoke emotion and watch as they move away from your mind. Repeat.

As you breathe, say this mantra: I allow thoughts to pass through my mind as sounds pass through my ears, naturally.

breathing practices reveal we are more
than our thoughts and patterns

Day 129
Number One

Treat yourself like your best friend.

We often have so much love and compassion to share yet forget to give the same to ourselves.

For today, consider all the well wishes you would send to a friend who was struggling, and return those well wishes onto yourself.

As you inhale and exhale, name the gifts you wish to give yourself. Breathing in: I am happy. Breathing out: I am unconditional love. Breathing in: I am confident. Breathing out: I am peace.

be compassionate with
number one—yourself

Day 130
Mantra: The Sacred Language of Sanskrit

At the core of mantra is the foundation of faith traditions, scriptures, and prayers.

Mantras have the power to alter life by supporting changing habits. They are the quiet healers, spoken in a whisper or in the silent speech of the mind. It can take months for the mantra to have an effect… to imprint on the body, mind, and soul. Or it can take an instant.

there is sacred power in the ritual of voice

Day 131
Once Upon a Week

Choose one self-loving mantra. Incorporate it into your internal dialogue—one mantra for a full week.

When it feels like a certain mantra is providing benefits, switch it up. Mantras are meant to suit your needs and personality, just as your internal dialogue is unique to you.

When you find a mantra that resonates, you will feel its vibrational strength to build confidence and love.

I am enough
I am abundant

Day 132
Superpower

Yoga is all about the power of prana, life force energy. Breath is the ultimate prana. It is what keeps us alive. It is also one of the only autonomous functions of the body that we also have the power to consciously control. Your breath is an incredible power.

breathing = living
mindful breathing = living large

Day 133
I Love Breath

Yoga will teach you to fall in love with your breath as you focus your attention and energy on this vital force of the body. Learning to control your breath can drastically affect your mood, energy, and life. Fall in love with your breath and watch your world transform.

Can you feel the pause at the end of your exhale? Enjoy that pause.

transformations happen through love

Day 134
Hatha

All is magic; all has meaning. Even if you don't see it now, you will one day. It will all make sense. It's not for nothing that you are here. It is everything that you are.

Every breath counts. Every single act in your life has richness and purpose. Without meaning, without truth, without love… it's a downward spiral into senselessness, sensationalism, and show.

In Sanskrit, hatha means: 'ha' for sun and 'tha' for moon.

Breathe today as if every inhale is sunlight, every exhale moonlight.

every breath is fresh, every breath is new

Day 135
Breathtaking Beauty

You have a choice about the kind of life you lead. You can let your environment dictate your experience, which means unless you solve all the problems of every person with whom you interact, you will always face some unhappiness. Or you can take control over your own experience of life. Buddhists suggest a middle path as the way to the pleasantness we all want, which means less time spent suffering.

Achieving more pleasantness is to come back to your breath over and over. Your breath and pleasant experiences are always available.

Can you feel the expanding sensations of the inhale and the contracting sensations of the exhale?

each time we come back to the breath we develop focus, concentration, and awareness

Day 136
Patient Pacing

Through the persistent effort to gain a deeper and more honest self-knowledge—and at the same time be in more generous and open communication with others—we create the conditions for transcendent insight to manifest in our experience.

If we want progress, we must focus on the inward and outward. That means: daily meditation—steadily, persistently, and patiently working on our minds to change unskillful into skillful mental states.

We must practice generosity constantly in our actions, words, and thoughts, always bringing ourselves back to the spirit of kindness when we gravitate towards selfishness and fear.

kind, slow, and steady triumphs
over any other pace

Day 137
Breath Speak

We've reached a day and age where showing emotional vulnerability can be viewed as a positive rather than a negative quality.

As you breathe today, can you bring a voice to what you've been keeping silent in your body?

People are becoming more aware and accepting of empathy and sensitivity. We are being encouraged to talk about our feelings, to seek help, and to connect with others. Gone are the days of keeping everything bottled up inside to suffer alone.

We're paying a price either way, so let's become more creative instead of a passive piece of creation.

breath is conversation
the universe is listening

Day 138
Holding Your Breath

Relationships are fluid just as the inhale-exhale cycle is fluid. This is just the way it is. Elation and unhappiness both show up, even in happy relationship. Thus, it is uncomfortable.

How can you breathe in the glory of your relationships and exhale the rigid thinking that causes you and your partner suffering?

Can you allow the breath to hold you both in the safety of a warm container of love?

breath is safety
I am safe

Day 139
Shine

Just as the suffering is present in every cell of our body, so are the seeds of awakened understanding and happiness handed down to us from our ancestors. We simply must nurture them.

We can bring light to our lives with mindfulness. That is the switch to reach for in the darkness. Mindfulness is the space between feeling and responding to feeling. Every day we can practice turning on that light.

breath is illumination

Day 140
Once Upon a Long Time Ago

Maybe you had a disappointment in your childhood that you've carried around for decades. Perhaps the way you were raised was less than ideal or something harmful that shaped your life. Maybe your disappointment is more recent: loss of a loved one, a failed relationship, or a major disease. No matter how disappointing or horrible it was, it is over now.

Like a tree that grows on the side of a mountain and is bent and shaped by heavy winds, you have been formed as you now are by this and other events of your life.

Let the experience go, allow it to have its death in the flow of time, for it is a natural part of time. Allow its death to be the fertilizer for what you cultivate in the life that it has left you. Breathe in and out, accepting and letting flow. Your breath can handle anything.

breath is your solace and shelter

Day 141
Hush...ush...ssh

We are self-healing metta human beings—we have just forgotten that. When we quiet the mind and use breath as the foundation for awakening, we stop doing and we become the healing. Take a deep inhale through the nose, down into the belly and slowly exhale through the mouth. Repeat this multiple times, when you're in the car, the office, standing in line, and feel the anxiety lessen.

Each day, as you practice, the body creates new pathways using your highest potential. You will naturally find yourself becoming a more relaxed person.

the body needs to move
and the mind needs stillness

Day 142
Breathing In, Breathing Out

Yoga is self discovery. The longest journey of any person is the journey inward.
   With each inhale say to yourself: I calm my body and mind.
   With each exhale say to yourself: I smile.

life requires great levels of patience

Day 143
Untapped Resources

The most difficult days can be the most fulfilling classrooms. The most challenging situations can become the most amazing teachers. Trust the process. Trust yourself. Rise from your darkness until you can kiss the sky.

Start construction now. Begin building the cathedral of you in this moment. All that is necessary for that first stone is to use your breath. One breath at a time builds the sanctuary and fortress of you. Build now to be ready for life's biggest moments.

you are so much more than you think you are

Day 144
Earth Breath

Reiki is a modality of energy healing. Practitioners use hands-on healing which originates from universal energy.

The practitioner acts as a vessel for the life energy (chi) to flow through, so that the reiki client can receive this energy.

Trust that the healing vibrations will go exactly where you need them. Bask in this glory. As you feel your breath, feel the whole universe in each.

the word earth is inside the word breath

Day 145
The Power of Love

As with a treasure behind a locked door, we can find the key that allows us to open the door of love. Love is like a muscle that can be strengthened through practice. As you sit in stillness today, let love be the energy you feel in your body, then, with each exhale, send this love out to the world.

love is breath, breath is love

Day 146
Grand Central Stations

Chakra is a Sanskrit word meaning wheel or disc. Chakras are points of the spiritual body that serve as the entry and exit points of our aura. These centers of energy are responsible for controlling our temperament, mood, and overall body health. They do so by receiving, assimilating, and expressing lifeforce energy, prana. Prana is ultimate, pure healing energy which is all around and within us to keep us healthy and vibrant.

pure lifeforce energy is active within us all

Day 147
Turn on the Light

Without awareness, we remain unconscious.

With maturity, we come to realize that which is unconscious remains unfulfilled or unhealed.

Forces that remain outside awareness are constantly working to keep what is hidden in darkness.

If we want to wake what is hidden, we need to be courageous and turn our attention to it—become aware.

What can you turn attention to now?

waking is an inside job
with universal implications

Day 148
Trust the Journey

We may not know all the specifics of what will happen to us when, or where… yet we now trust in a process.

Trust and breath are a kind of love linked within our lifeforce.

To swim against our natural current is exhausting. Instead, choose to go with the flow.

Have you noticed you never quite get there and something else is always coming?

When we understand this pattern, we can accept we are fluid and always in process.

your destiny is sacred

Day 149
Be

True spiritual growth is as much about taking away or not doing as it is about having and doing. Loving includes tough choices like the pain of walking away when we're still in love. Trust the abundance of the universe. Walking away in love is love.

Have you noticed this?

Could you sacrifice a love for an abundant universe full of love?

With each breath, notice when you tend to hang on, use your exhale to practice letting go.

love is honesty

Pratyahara: The 5th Limb

"When we let go of the continual construction of a self or even the need to be a 'somebody,' then we are free to be who we are. When we are completely ourselves, we forget about needing to be the center of our perceptual world and thus we can take in others and our environment with greater sensitivity, compassion, and openness."
MICHAEL STONE, *THE INNER TRADITION OF YOGA: A GUIDE TO YOGA PHILOSOPHY FOR THE CONTEMPORARY PRACTITIONER*

Slowly, through practice, we tune into a place within us that exists beyond our senses. Sometimes it is challenging, yet it is a vital part of the eight limbs of yoga. The withdrawal of the senses is called pratyahara.

Pratyahara practice is essentially relevant now because we live in a world of overstimulation. We constantly receive input from devices, and we instinctively and instantly react. We have been pulled away from inner peace. We can end up reacting all day long.

Anything that shifts the focus from external noise to internal peaceful feelings is pratyahara.

Detoxing from media and creating space from things that work against us (think: toxins) will help us in our practice.

The Pratyahara Days

Day 150
Relaxation

Relaxation eases muscular and nervous tension, abstracts the senses from their objects, makes silence and concentration easy, and contributes to peace of mind. Relaxation provides an entry into the subconscious planes. When this happens, natural harmony between the body and the mind is revived and sustained. Consistent relaxation practice activates our natural relaxation response in the body. This is how we combat stress and find peace in the midst of chaos.

Can you include more relaxation for yourself in the day?

it is vital to water the
seeds of relaxation within you

Day 151
Wholeness

We do a lot of things that help us get what we want. The getting and wanting are aligned with ego. Ego is the small part of us that judges, criticizes, doubts, and fears. Ego is always in a state of lack and dissatisfaction. Pratyahara opens us to receive the opposite of ego, the love beyond the lack.

all we seek is within

Day 152
Your Own Umbrella

What you let into your mind is dependent solely on you.

At best, the actions of others will not distract you from your focus. At worst, the actions of others will knock you off your path.

Who are you? Are you strong enough to stand on your own two feet?

What do you do daily to stay grounded? (Examples: exercise, read, walk, practice yoga, meditate.)

Can you notice the pulling sensation in your body that tells you it's time for quietness?

When we take care of ourselves, we can be aware of the oncoming waves and be strong enough to manage the stress by responding skillfully. When we ignore body, mind, and intuitive self, the water comes, we get soaked, and it takes a long time to dry. Either way, we are learning.

experiences are classrooms

Day 153
Stillness in the Storm

We are busy people. The daily pressures of work, children, finances, and chores can be overwhelming, leaving us anxious, frustrated, even depressed. To soothe our negative feelings, we may turn to shopping, drinking, anger, or another unhealthy habit.

Can we possibly find peace in life's chaos?

We can. It starts by recognizing how stressed we really are and the effect it has on our mental and physical well-being. Then, with this awareness, we can find ways to bring calm into our lives. Some simple ways include meditating, listening to music, getting a massage, enjoying a cup of hot tea or coffee, watching a sunset, taking a walk.

we are our own calm creators

Day 154
Forever Peace

Any activity that makes us happy and feel more relaxed helps bring peace in the moment. Now, what about creating lasting peace—the kind that gives us a sense of wellness and renewal?

Lasting peace is created from within. When we practice gratitude, when we affirm goodness and serve others and ourselves in a kindly way, we build lasting peace. When we forgive others, our truthful, loving self emerges, bringing a tranquil spirit. When we do all this, we become life- changers.

peace is within us

Day 155
Feeling Peace

Eventually, through yogic inner-peace practices, we begin to experience feelings as feelings—impersonal phenomena as opposed to feelings in the form of explosive dramas played out by storytelling. Feeling is the key to the present moment. It anchors us in experience. Observing patterns of our feelings, we can attach less stories to them.

Can you notice and allow feelings to arise and pass in your body today?

Notice where you tend to attach stories to the feelings. Repeat: I am safe to experience peace.

stay in the moment, for the moment is peace

Day 156
Be Proud

Human beings have spent much time and energy over millennia improving external conditions in their search for happiness and peace.

The result is that while some of their wishes have been fulfilled, human suffering has continued to increase while the experience of happiness and peace is decreasing. This clearly shows that we need to find a true method for gaining pure happiness and freedom from misery.

Reflecting daily and inquiring within is one method to connect deeply with your inner kingdom of solutions, abundance, knowledge, and skills. Be proud of yourself for taking this time for you today. What does it feel like to be proud of yourself?

it is never too late, never too dark;
you are an infinite spark

Day 157
Little Secret

Conscious connection to something allows us to feel and experience that thing, person, or event. Yoga connects us to joy, bliss, and fulfillment. Awareness is the secret of yoga.

How can you bring connection alive today? Keep a loving mantra (I am love) as an inner secret.

follow the bliss

Day 158
Continuity

In the Buddhist tradition, the terms "loving-kindness" and "compassion" refer to qualities of the mind and heart, and to specific meditation practices that help develop these qualities. Loving-kindness and compassion greatly enhance the ability to stay aware in meditation practice and in daily life. These qualities can be difficult to develop in any depth; for some, they can be hard to understand. Yet, fostering their development is essential for spiritual maturation.

How can you define loving-kindness and compassion today?

as in yoga, so in daily life

Day 159
Wanderlust

We determine our lives by the actions we take when we are unsure of something. Curating our curiosity to make it a soul-seeking adventure can remove the element of fear (of ego).

How do you react when you are not certain?

What stories do you tell yourself in these moments?

there is treasure in the unknown

Day 160
Learning Journey

Be gone, myth of the hero who is always right. Away with you, perfectionist who we know will never be satisfied. Live fully in your imperfect self. That way life will experience you—as well as how you experience life. Let the learning be a two-way street so all can evolve. Let's celebrate the imperfect, the mistakes, and carry the glory of being human on our shoulders.

sacred are the learners

Day 161
Mantric

Here are some effective mantras:

I have much to celebrate.

I am kind to myself.

Om mani padme hum (a Tibetan mantra which means "Hail the jewel in the lotus").

Om namah shivaya (known as the Shree Shivapanchakshari mantra, it calls upon Lord Shiva who is responsible for the destruction of evil).

Take notice the connection to the spiritual world you feel when repeating a mantra.

life is an en-chant-ing experience

Day 162
Boomerang

Intention is powerful. What you send out energetically returns to you. Whether you refer to this as the laws of karma, the rules of physics, or simple cause and effect, it is undeniable that intention holds strong value.

give back, give present, give forward

Day 163
A Spark Is Light

We need to balance the light and darkness within us. Far too often, we fear the dark and adore only the light.

When we acknowledge that darkness has a place in life—a silent time-out to allow the soul to grow or experience sorrow—then we can welcome the light from a place of having become friends with our inner darkness.

closed eyes can help us be
aware of the dark, and opening
our eyes invites light; we are both

Day 164
Impermanence

Autumn immerses us in impermanence. We've found the buds, touched the flowers, and then comes the golden, colourful season when the leaves fall and bare branches remind us of the immortal nature of all things.

Rest and renewal, the heavily golden tones at sunset, the crisp air floating beneath an eternal sun flame. The embrace of a young friend. Temporary, fleeting, the season to harvest all that is goodness and joy, reminding us of the life cycle in which we are all golden participants.

we are all passing through life

Day 165
Respond Softly

Teachings require logic to parse. In the heat of an emotional exchange, you may not have the luxury of logic because logic requires time to process with an unbiased mind. Pressure creates a crisis in which you will likely not have time to think, only to react.

What is needed is a well-honed, quickly deployed skill—something short, easy to use, and effective—that gives enough space and helps remove bias. One of these skills is the Third Moment Method, which we will explore over the next few days.

respond to crisis with the same softness
as a mother tends to her baby

Day 166
1st of 3 Moments: Sensing

The Third Moment Method is a practical tool that in many ways embodies the core of Buddhist practice, in that it helps us slow down and create emotional distance in the moment.

Life is composed of a series of experiences; each of these experiences can be broken into three moments.

The first moment: sensing.

The eyes, ears, and nose perceive input. Sensing is effortless—hardwired into our system. The time between a sound reaching the ear and the perception of that sound seems immediate.

In this moment—the first moment—if someone says the word "lemon," the word has been heard, and it is without recognition of what that sound means.

we are amazing, sentient, feeling beings

Day 167
2ⁿᵈ of 3 Moments: Arising

In the second moment: arising, we recognize the sound—or other sensation—and we have an instant, subconscious response, classifying it as good, bad, or neutral. This, too, is automatic, based on prior experience: memories and understanding stemming from conditioned cultural beliefs, religious creeds, and linguistic perceptions.

It happens so quickly that we may even think it is part of the first moment. We have a physical manifestation of thought as the body responds to positive, negative, or neutral input.

For example, someone is describing a juicy lemon they've just sliced. We connect the sound made by the combination of letter-sounds in "lemon" to an idea stored in memory. It evokes a shape, a color, a scent, a taste. Memory invites an emotional response. Maybe we enjoy lemons and instantly crave the flavour, or we don't enjoy them and cringe from the imagined sourness.

Either way, we are in recognition.

our senses serve us

Day 168
3rd of 3 Moments: Reacting

In the Third Moment: reacting, there is the choice of reacting with acceptance.

Our reaction may be mental, verbal, or physical. If we have classified something as good, we are drawn to it, even though it may not be beneficial. If we have classified something as bad, we push it away, sometimes with more force than needed. In either case, we may do a lot of damage that will need to be undone later.

For example, think of the lemon in a different context. What if the mechanic says your brand-new car is a lemon? How would you feel? What might you say to the person who advised you to buy it?

The Third Moment provides the space to determine how we would like to respond. Our response might be reactive or it might be creative—gentler in a thoughtful, slow evaluation.

each moment is an opportunity
to be creative and kind

Day 169
Spacing

Cultivating awareness of the Three Moments is a Zen practice. Practicing this allows for valuable space to evaluate and/or curate a response to whatever situation is arising.

You can use this space to respond to how you want to be in the now.

you can contribute to kindness
and compassion in the world

Day 170
Practicing the Third Moment

Aim to observe emotion today in a unique, determined way. The moment an emotion rises, pause… close your eyes and breathe. Take note of the emotion. Can you notice it before it can connect with thought? See it for what it is, as a sensation and not what it becomes after it connects with thought or a story.

pause and observe emotions
in the body, as clouds float through the sky

Day 171
Prayer

Prayer is an action towards the divine life you are seeking and creating. Pray often for answers, to forgive and to align with your purest compassionate self.

Bless this world and all those afflicted with despair and doubt, show them light and love. May they see glory in the eyes of strangers. Be with us all today as we grow to becoming closer to our Father and Mother God and Goddess. I believe in love. I believe in faith. Make me an instrument of kindred peace. Have mercy on my soul and forgive me my sins.

May I be better tomorrow than today.

we can bring our inner peace
to any experience

Day 172
Feel the Feeling and Let It Go

You may be tempted to trace the source of your emotion. Sure, that might be logical, but it is not always helpful. Rather than focussing on who did what, focus on your actual experience and try to feel it directly. Feel your emotion as if it is an inflated balloon, filling your insides. Don't pay attention to the balloon itself but to what's inside it. What does it feel like? No rationalizing. No reasoning. What is at the very core of the balloon? Feel the feeling—and now let it go.

it's productive to feel our experiences
and then let them go; there is more

Day 173
Vibes In and Out

We do not have to label or relabel our emotions. Instead, we can understand that a specific emotion does not exist in the way we believe it does—as something fixed and solid. Every emotion vibrates differently. Every emotion is a vibrational pattern.

Over time, as awareness grows, we can begin to feel ease, maybe even joy.

perception and perspective are fluid

Day 174
Receiving

In yoga, we learn to become intimate with our emotions. When we open up the space between receiving and reaction, we can come to truly understand our emotions. Acceptance of our emotions opens us to joyfully experience life. There is more love when we are not clinging to one emotion.

we are more than our emotions—we are love

Day 175
Shakti

Many times we fill the divine space of our mind with unnecessary stories (thoughts, responses, and perceptions). Mindful living—in love with the universe—involves tuning into the energetic movement called the Tao, or, in Sanskrit, Shakti. It is also known as the cosmic intention or destiny.

What do you feel destined to achieve or accomplish?

a naturally intelligent life-force moves and compels you

Day 176
Four Noble Truths

The four noble truths in Buddhism are the truth of suffering, the truth of the cause of suffering, the truth of the end of suffering, and the truth of the path that leads to the end of suffering.

Buddhism suggests that escape from these is possible through nirvana.

How can you describe your definition of nirvana?

the sages have much to teach us

Day 177
Transcend - Dance

There needs to be a constant movement between going deeper into the inward-looking aspect and being ever more expansive in the outward-looking aspect. This is the creative tension of the spiritual life which eventually leads to a transcendence of inward and outward.

we are always in motion
life is a dance

Day 178
Metta

Change often seems inconvenient at its best and traumatic at its worst. To change is to move beyond current attachments… and that is difficult because our attachments are what give us security and stability.

Through our spiritual practices we develop an inner stability and security. When we become intimate with uncertainty and impermanence and use our spiritual practices to stabilize, we are reminded what metta is: positive energy and kindness. We need positive practices to balance the negative we hear all around us.

turning love inward provides solid ground

Day 179
Calming

The main reason it is so difficult to be patient with others is because we experience ourselves as the centre of the universe. From this standpoint we can get hurt and upset and angry when others don't seem to go along with our centralized version of us.

Yoga doesn't change these viewpoints, it transforms the person who sees. Close your eyes in order to see. Can you loosen your grip on any stories and speech with "I," "me," and "mine"?

we is me
me is we

Day 180
Thoughtfulness

In order to develop patience towards others, we must go beyond any selfishness and begin to see that real self-interest includes the interests of others. This requires imagination and a willingness to question our anger and indignation.

Behind anger there is love. There are people awaiting your care. Ask often, how can I serve?

to serve others is to serve me

Day 181
Depth Wish

Expecting relationships to be comfortable is what makes them uncomfortable.

At the root of discomfort is our wish for comfort. We think everything will be fine if we can only find that special person. Then, when we do find that someone special, we decide everything is not fine. All the fears we have not handled flow into the relationship dynamic.

How does any relationship thrive? Those that flow do so when blame is not assigned and we are kind to each other as we are being tossed about or smoothing our rough edges against each other.

What would it be like if, instead of wishing for comfort, we wished for depth?

What if the first thing we brought to our disconnects was curiosity rather than judgment?

kindness is the balm for pain,
and the salve in relationships

Day 182
Proactive

It's human nature to have negativity bias: we're more sensitive to what's going wrong than what's going right. It's how we're hardwired, a means to stay safe. We can and will rewire. Every yogic practice is like adding software.

Life is about more than just being safe. At least I want it to be. I want to focus more on what I love than what I fear. I want to be proactive, not just reactive. I want to wake up every day and be the good that happens to someone else instead of just playing defense to prevent bad from happening to me.

What do you wish to impress upon others? Ask yourself: "What good can I do next?"

choose love each day

Day 183
Sacred Heart

Within every human there is love in its purest form. This is where we store the wishes we place upon coins before tossing them into fountains. It's the place where we hold memories that make our eyes sparkle and our hearts beat with joy. The place inside us where we dream big and live fearlessly. It is a love for us and a love for all life.

If anything defines us, it is love. Each of us has the heart of the world. Can you feel the heartbeat of the world is the same as the heartbeat in your chest?

our heart is a home of love

Day 184
Majestic

While life is a mystery, it does not have to be a dramatic, scary one. We can accept that disappointment will be part of our learning, and that disappointment can be reframed into growth, then we need not hope for the best. We will be delivered a majestic mix of sacred mystery.

opening to mystery
cultivates wonder, awe, and curiosity

Day 185
Put Forth

Most people want the rewards of consciousness without the hard work of consciousness. The hard work of consciousness requires developing a daily spiritual practice that allows us to review where we are investing our energy each day.

Each morning and each evening we have a choice: do we invest our energy into fears and anxieties or do we invest our energy into aligning with spiritual truth or love?

where our focus goes, our energy flows

Day 186
Centred

Think back to a time when you were feeling stressed or afraid. What physical reactions did you experience?

Tense muscles, rapid breathing, sweating palms, and a racing heart are all common reactions to a stressful situation.

Now, imagine all of these feelings are the result of energy flowing through your body.

Centring is training your mind to redirect energy to the centre of your body, or to your breath. Centring is establishing a sense of inner calm.

centre yourself several times a day

Day 187
Art of Self-Care

If you are not taking care of yourself, how can you give your best self to others?
Self-care is healthcare, and it is an essential part of us. Make a list of how you currently take care of yourself. What can you add to the list?

self-care is necessary self-love

Day 188
Sharing Is Caring

How many of us have the courage on a daily basis—or multiple times a day—to go and stand in front of a room full of people and open ourselves up and pour ourselves out for no better purpose than to foster healing and positivity in the lives of those around?

How can you share your purpose and kindness with others? What can you offer to others?

bravery is sourced from love
courage calls us to share

Day 189
Starlight

You are the sun and the moon, the stars and the earth, and the roots of the trees combined together in a unique energy called life. You illuminate galaxies. There is beauty in the way you move through this world. Do you know this? Believe it.

Take a pause to realize your value and your wonder today.

What does knowing and believing this goodness feel like inside you?

How can you share this with the world?

you are a transformational artist
you are complete light

Day 190
Hidden Depths

Without awareness, we remain unconscious. As we gain maturity, we begin to understand that what is in the unconscious remains unhealed. As it turns out, forces outside of conscious awareness work ceaselessly to keep what is hidden in darkness. This is referred to as our shadow self. We are unaware of the shadow as we are unaware of darkness.

To awaken what is hidden, we must first turn our attention to it.

Let us awaken with an attitude not to blame or shame, rather to suspend judgment and meet these hidden depths of ourselves with compassion.

What have you suppressed?

where there is light of awareness,
shadows disappear...without light, they grow

Day 191
Set Free

Forgiveness is a loving practice, for yourself. This spiritual practice releases all that is false and blows sand off the mirror of our inner beauty.

We need positive practices to balance the negative we hear all around us.

There's nothing more compassionate than forgiving yourself or someone else for things they've done or not done.

forgiving ourselves means loving ourselves—
forgiving others means loving others

Day 192
Define Your Dreams

The universe is one big opportunity machine.

Everything that could contribute to our happiness is either right in front of us or speeding at us.

What is the biggest, wildest dream inside of you right now?

dwell in infinite possibilities

Day 193
Management

Every thought you have is based on your perception, your angle of how you see the world. Therefore, the world is an accumulation of your thoughts. If you want to change the world—your world—it is through changing your thoughts. You *can* manage your thoughts and you *can* manage your emotions.

live free of clinging thoughts
in order to love freely

Dharana: The 6th Limb

"When thoughts come up, touch them very lightly, like a feather touching a bubble. Let the whole thing be soft and gentle, but at the same time precise."
PEMA CHÖDRÖN, THE WISDOM OF NO ESCAPE: AND THE PATH OF LOVING-KINDNESS

When we focus on one thing, all other things—little things, big things, medium things—fall away. We might be lost in sketching, or reading an amazing story, or preparing a lesson plan, and we experience a kind of peace.

This is what dharana is: an intentional focus of mind.

Dharana is where we move to a deeper part of yoga, by bringing consciousness to a single point of concentration. When we practice dharana, we focus on a chakra, or a part of the body, or we could choose an external image like a picture or an item of interest. The purpose is to concentrate the mind.

Dharana practice develops a container or a space to hold longer periods of meditation.

The Dharana Days

Day 194
Sow Love

Your heart is a garden, a magical place which, when tenderly cared for turns seeds into trees, berry bushes, wildflowers, and herbs.

Focus today on what seeds you plant in your heart. Are there wholesome seeds you can add?

cultivate love, joy, peace
you are divine grace

Day 195
Wellspring of Joy

Deep inside you is a place where happiness is born. We access it by easing our minds, having a positive—and realistic—outlook, by carrying out genuine acts of kindness towards others. Happiness feeds our courage, thus, when we face difficulties, we are brave enough to deal with them.

If we want to be happy then, as Buddha said, we need to tame our minds.

courage and kindness intertwine
we are divine

Day 196
Sumeru

A mala string contains 108 beads. One of the beads is called a sumeru, or head bead. The beads are used to focus on prayer, meditation, chant or mantra, and to count in sets. Sumeru marks the beginning and the end of the mala.

supportive tools bathed in
centuries of wisdom are available to us

Day 197
No Time

We may think we have the time. We may believe that we have forever to do certain things, pursue creative avenues, or even tell someone they are loved. Because of that thinking, we wait—we put off the being and the doing.

Awareness of impermanence can free us from all that waiting and can help us realize how important it is to find the courage to experience life in the here and now.

impermanence, thank you kindly

Day 198
Once Upon a Practice

Unless you're lost in a fairy tale, the path to true love can be a challenge, yet it can also be exhilarating, progressive, and worthwhile. Fairy tales make us think of the magic that freezes the first kiss moments.

Outside the fairy tale, we can feel sad that first kiss moments don't last forever. There is no escape from inevitable change. When challenges arise, it is our practice and recalling that this too shall pass, which will help us move through.

the happily ever after is in the
transcending—we can write
a love story of life

Day 199
Rhythmic Channel

Mantras provide a point of focus a rhythm that makes it simple for the mind and body to embrace. Mantra brings a wandering mind back to point, and its internal sound vibration creates a channel for energy to flow in and out. When a person knows the meaning of their mantra, there is a deeper impact.

mantras are soul-powered rhythm and meaningful lyric which resonate for a higher purpose

Day 200
Practical Magic

You likely have a friend or family member that lets the negative self-talk overpower their positive, self-loving thoughts. It is so painful to watch them beat themselves up, but we all do it from time to time.

If ever you feel yourself being less than kind to yourself, try one of these self-loving mantras to regain confidence and move forward. You can focus on the first phrase, memorize the entire thought, or modify one of the below to your specific needs.

I love myself. I am a unique spirit. I am completely worthy of love. I am worthy of being loved and respected by others. I am perfectly imperfect. I am flawlessly flawed. I am goodness.

words are powerful forces
for unconditional love

Day 201
Great Story

Be courageous enough to tell your story—a good story—about the beauty that has touched you, about the love you have given and received, about forgiveness, happiness, and the lessons compassion gifts you.

embrace the unique greatness
of your life story

Day 202
Buddha Nature

If I am, for example, suffering with a debilitating disease, or paralyzed by grief, then I will probably see myself as not being normal. I will feel there is something wrong with me.

According to Buddha, whose teachings say the nature of life is suffering, it is being genuinely happy and healthy that is unusual. There is a level of unease with us all the time—such is the nature of life.

Once we observe deeply, we see that every living thing has suffered or will suffer. We can use our awareness of impermanence to engage in the flow of life.

we are created to handle
and transcend great storms

Day 203
Higher Vibration

We have hurt others by being dishonest, going behind their backs, speaking ill of them, or confronting them in anger. We have been hurt by others in all these ways as well. It is the way of humans; we are vibrating beings. When we dedicate ourselves to supporting goodness as a practice and kindness as a way of life, then we can advance beyond—vibrate higher—than the former behaviours. All this requires forgiveness of others and of ourselves. By forgiving, the mind gets calm and we rid ourselves of negative feelings.

Do you have someone you would love to forgive?

forgiveness allows us to transform life
and raise our vibration

Day 204
Every Moment Is Fresh

There are times when we experience events and plead with the universe for the moment to never end. Of course, it will. Everything is living—moments, the air, the ground… and everything living also transforms—dies, dissolves, changes. This thing called life and this concept called living is so wonderous it is a moment-by-moment spectacular performance of now. It is so magnificent it is almost incomprehensible.

see the wonder in every moment, in every
blink of an eye, in every breath

Day 205
Levels of Experiences

For a long time, linguistic folklore said that the Inuit people had fifty words for snow. Because the climate of the arctic dominates their life, they do have an abundance of words which describe snow.

It is like this in Buddhist thought; there are many words for, or connected to, suffering. Among them, somewhere in the hierarchy of expression, there is "plain old suffering" (not a technical term), the kind we experience when someone dies, or we become ill, or something precious is lost, or when circumstance doesn't break in our favour. All human beings experience these things.

Can you open to experiencing the depths of your suffering in relation to the height of your love?

each person's experiences of suffering
are unique to that person

Day 206
The Suffering of Suffering

The suffering of suffering represents the additional discomfort or pain we tag to regular suffering.

The suffering of suffering arises from the stories we tell ourselves and the incorrect judgments we make from those stories.

Suffering "A" is unavoidable. Suffering "B" is optional.

The Buddhist eightfold path is a way to understand our journey of life.

love and relationships are profound paths

Day 207
Intimately You

When we are connected to others we can come to know our patterns, see where we are, and become better people. Yet, to connect intimately to others we need to have done some inner work and know ourselves. It is a circle, a continuum of growth.

Each relationship is a chance to continue becoming the best version of you. Keep going.

relationships are sacred
everything and everyone is connected

Day 208
If Only

Life can be hard. You finally get what you want in your career, or in a relationship, or a lifestyle, yet there are still all these problems you had assumed would go away if only this or that happened. Sometimes you will gradually realize that the thing you always wanted is never going to happen—having a child or a loving spouse, making peace with a difficult parent, finding creative expression, or getting economic freedom. It's not that there aren't lots of good times too; it's that the disappointments can loom so large.

What are the stories you are attaching when the emotions arise?

Be aware that you can create less suffering and new stories for yourself. This is self-love.

Reframing can reduce the symptoms of suffering. Awareness is one of the first steps to reducing your suffering.

you can suffer less because your mind can
create a love story out of any experience

Day 209
Sacrifice

The person who wishes to alleviate suffering—who wishes to fix the flaws of being; who wants to bring about the best of all possible futures; who wants to create heaven on earth—will make the greatest of sacrifices, of self and child, of everything that is loved, to live a life aimed at the good.

If you have felt an urge to speak a truth you are called to speak, please speak it now. The universe needs you now.

when you give up something
the universe brings you something greater

Day 210
School for Self

A relationship is a mirror. In every moment, one individual reveals the other. Close relationships are clear mirrors.

Consider what is stirring emotion in you about the other. Could this be a lesson for you also? Could you give this away? Sometimes all that is missing in a relationship is what you are not giving.

relationships are classrooms;
private and self-directed learning

Day 211
Infinite Sparkle

This cosmos is our mirror into everything that happens deep in our soul and heart. Our soul is sparkling like thousands of diamonds that catch the light. During the nights of new moons, our hearts are going to be opened, and seeds will be planted. We are going to enter a new domain of comprehension and wisdom.

Are you open to receive the universal gifts coming to you?

What can you let go of to create room for abundance that is larger than your thoughts?

the map of the universe is within

Day 212
Peaceful Path

The key is to find peace in our hearts even in those moments that bring us to our knees.

The trick is to find strength within our hopelessness, and to find faith when we've lost our willingness to believe.

We may see these moments as our spiritual test, yet are they not really our own spiritual awakening?

Keep this in your awareness today: "I can relax amid any chaos."

relaxing amid chaos, learning not to panic
is the spiritual path

Day 213
Always Ask

Reflect on what arises when you ask yourself: "What could I do, that I would do, to make life a little better?"

You can choose. Choose joy. Choose love. Choose truth. Choose heart. Choose forgiveness.

in asking, we receive—
and the answer is always love

Day 214
Multidimensional

We are multidimensional beings who have power beyond any power we've been told we have. The things we can learn are immensely more powerful than the simple tools we think are all we have at our disposal.

We are powerful beings, and together we can heal this world. If we tune into higher dimensions, we can feel the light of higher consciousness. We can be certain it exists energetically, and experience a knowingness that it will manifest into form.

we are super conscious,
metta human beings who can heal

Day 215
Movement

We are each summoned to do the incredibly challenging work of ultimate self transformation.

What is your work? How are you transforming? What does that look like?

we are dynamic, active, energetic beings

Day 216
Monitor

Today, pay close attention: are you following the gripping energy of fear or the liberating energy of love? Where do you get stuck in either? Could you dance between the two?

the way to freedom is through love—
and love is always available

Dhyana: the 7th Limb

"Every moment is incredibly unique and fresh, and when we drop
into the moment, as meditation allows us to do, we learn how to truly
taste this tender and mysterious life that we share together."
PEMA CHÖDRÖN, HOW TO MEDITATE

The word dhyana comes from the Sanskrit word dhyai, which means: to think of.

It is in the deepest parts of the mind we find self-knowledge. We get there through meditation—deep concentration. This is the way we find a union with source.

Most yoga practitioners are doing yoga to feel good and learn more about themselves, and to find moments of peace during busy times—this makes finding permanent bliss a bit more than we bargained for. Even unreachable.

The purpose of meditation is to relax and free the mind, especially the memory, which is the hardest segment to quiet. Memory is continually feeding us stories of our past and contributing to conjuring up what might happen in the future, limited to only past memories.

The mind, including memory, can sit for a moment, then another moment, and then many moments strung together until it is much more than a moment.

Bliss is achievable. We can condition the mind through consistent meditation training.

Today, for a few minutes, tune out of all external sounds—turn off your notifications, set a timer for five minutes, then shut off the playlist and sit with whatever arises with an attitude of kindness. Find the power in silence. You are more than your thoughts.

The Dhyana Days

Day 217
Insecurity

When I'm insecure, I act in ways I normally wouldn't.

I've asked myself if it was jealousy, though my beliefs are much stronger than that. I've asked myself if it was other people. Then I came to learn the answers are always "me."

Insecurity, you are a sneaky little problem-causing poison. I'm sure the roots of insecurity from my inner critic date back to my childhood. I've conquered self-worth, self-esteem, confidence. I know who I am. I thought I was pretty well balanced until night when the wind is knocked out of me.

I learned insecurity is caused by wanting permanence. We feel fear and insecurity when we are anxious about the root anchors of our life being unstable. In truth, one who understands impermanence knows nothing is permanent. At a deep level, we must see how resting on inherently unstable emotional platforms and expecting stability is folly. There is no easy cure for this. We must, at the very least, learn to dissociate our identity and sense of self from worldly factors such as a job, a relationship, a degree, a house. This can be done through any of the several forms of meditation and/or yoga practices.

our yoga, meditation, and stories are essential curriculum to healing

Day 218
Remember Death

Contemplation and meditation on death and impermanence are a part of Buddhism because we are all always dying.

Recognizing the shortness of life, and how precious it is, will help us live in a meaningful way.

Through understanding the process of death, even familiarizing ourselves with it, we can reduce our fear at the time of death, therefore creating a meaningful rebirth.

What would you do if today was your last day?

live and love each day as if it is the last

Day 219
Don't Believe Everything You Think

When we hit a snag in life, encounter a difficulty, have to deal with a problem, if we can apply a positive and peaceful mind, there would be less drama, shorter-term problems and, ultimately, fewer snags. If we treat challenges as opportunities to grow, we vibrate higher and attract people, places, and things that vibe high.

freedom from problems requires
learning to control the mind

Day 220
Heart Wisdom

It's been said that the furthest distance in the universe is from the head to the heart.

Despite that great inferred distance, it is in stillness that we find this path. It is in the quiet space that we can get out of our heads and connect more deeply with ourselves, thereby allowing ourselves to be open to the possibilities when they arrive.

the quieter the mind, the louder the heart

Day 221
Sitting Still

Meditation is an incredibly useful tool to bridge the head and heart connection.

Consistently carving out time in the day for quiet, then getting quiet allows us to find peace and connect with our nature, stillness. For today, try saying this to yourself: "I don't have to have all the answers or know what is going to happen next."

it is a gift to the world when we
sit in our silence

Day 222
Mantra Is

Mantra is more than a repeated phrase. Mantra vibrates throughout the body, focusses the mind, and transports positivity into the mind.

A mantra provides an array of spiritual, mental, and physical healing for the practitioner. For example: *I am enough.*

Choose a mantra for today. Repeat it while feeling your whole being absorbed in the resonance of each word, and allow your throat to be the vessel through which that energy kisses the air as it leaves your physical body.

vibrations are energy; the higher
intent of the energy, the more sacred

Day 223
Mantra Meaning

When people think of mantra meditation, the word "om" comes to mind. Om is a Hindu word that means, "it is" or "to become."

What is important during the chanting of om is the vibration it creates in the body. These vibrations create neuro-linguistic effects. These effects induce a sense of calm. They often help people with serious illness, and they provide to those who feel a sense of hopelessness. They gift fullness to those who feel lack.

full participation in chanting allows
rhythm and energy to transform us

Day 224
Double Duty

When the meaning of a mantra is known to the person meditating, psycho-linguistic effects are added to the neuro-linguistic effects. These are effective in goal-oriented meditation. Someone who is trying to overcome an addiction can find this beneficial. The same is true for someone starting a new habit. The meaning of the mantra imprints on the subconscious so when the person comes out of the meditative state, the mantra is still working.

the subconscious is a wise,
all-knowing aspect of each of us

Day 225
Insight Meditation

Many people practice a Buddhist form of meditation called vipassana, or insight meditation. In this particular practice, one first learns to stabilize the mind by focussing on a single object, such as the breath. Once concentration is strong, the mind is allowed to move as it chooses while the individual remains mindful of the process so as not to get lost in thought.

Of course, we do get lost in thoughts as well as feelings and body sensations, over and over again, but each time we stray, we correct and then return to awareness. Gradually the mind becomes much steadier. With a steady mind, insight arises.

mindfully we grow
insights can fuel our actions

Day 226
Spaciousness

Vipassana practice cultivates an awareness of spaciousness—all thoughts and feelings experienced without the mind contracting. This provides a sense of inner freedom. With the mind awake in this manner, we can more clearly see within. Insights arise and can guide us. We gain a sense of seeing things how they truly are, as nature: interconnected.

increased awareness and a quiet mind
is your birthright

Day 227
Journey Versus Destination

Another wise distinction that relates both to yoga practice and other aspects of life is understanding the difference between the journey and the destination. Our culture is compulsively fast paced and goal oriented. We insist on arriving at destinations.

However, there is nowhere to get to because we are already here—present on a journey.

life is a journey of love

Day 228
Using a Mala

A mala can be a beaded necklace or bracelet. If you have one, then you can hold it to use it, and if you don't have one, choose an image of one to look at. Use each bead to help focus your mind, you can repeat a mantra at each bead.

Learning to use a mala can be a wonderful way to deepen your meditation practice.

the wisdom of the ancients—
including their tools—
are connections to our present

Day 229
Labour of Love

Each time we return to breath and calm in meditation, we develop the mind. Throughout the day, outside meditation, the mindfulness we learn in meditation is with us, keeping us calm and focussed, helping us respond creatively and with less reactivity.

one of our greatest powers
is the power of focus

Day 230
Great Truth

It is the truth that burns bright in every human. It is the shift from fear to love. It is the loss of separation and the essential gain of oneness. The birth of omnipresence and all the powers and magic it contains within its glory. And it is the loss of who we thought we were and essentially all we ever thought at all.

If we so choose.

For no one is being told what to do.

We own the greatest power: the free will to choose what we will own up to.

However, truth does not change. It can expand to entail infinite beauties and mystical realms. The choice to see this as is, is up to whom we have become and wish to be.

Do you know who you are? Do you know who you want to be?

When we are able to answer these questions, we continue the journey and experience true fulfilment.

truth is as we are—
endless, abundant, infinite

Day 231
Being Peace

The more we practice, the more often we get to be in our enlightened mind. We come to realize that outside our practice we are still a little bit in practice, then a little bit more. Soon we are living in gratitude, rather than choosing a few moments of it. The same with peace. The same with quiet. Then, in our new way of being, rather than doing—as we find ourselves being more rather than doing more, we find clarity. We see the train tracks, rather than the horizon. We look out the window and notice what is right beside us, not what is up ahead. We begin to be the journey.

presence is peace, peace is presence

Day 232
Progress

Through the persistent effort to gain a deeper and more honest self-knowledge and, at the same time, be in more generous and open communication with others, we create the conditions for transcendent insight to manifest in our experience.

If we want to evolve in love, then we continuously need to trust in these two directions: the inward and outward. Daily meditation is required, steadily, persistently, and patiently working on our minds to change unskillful mental states into skillful mental states.

We must constantly practice generosity in our actions, words, and thoughts, always bringing ourselves back to the spirit of generosity when we gravitate towards selfishness and fear.

gratitude, gratitude, gratitude

Day 233
Beyond

You may have strong experiences in meditation from time to time, and they may give you faith that states of consciousness exist beyond what you usually experience. Please don't get distracted by these experiences or start to chase them. What is really important is whether you are kind and generous and truthful the rest of the time and whether your relations with others are becoming friendlier.

stay in the zone of truth

Day 234
Moving Relationships

Whether you are about to go on a blind date with someone you have never set eyes on or are upset with your partner of thirty years because they've done the thing they promised to never do, again, you are unable to find solid ground.

That means the security blanket of pleasantness has been shaken. Can you see this now as an element of the process of being in relationship? Can you be comfortable in uncertainty knowing it is moving through while happening for you?

relationships are an unsteady
and beautifully moving dance

Day 235
Strongly We Grow

Today, in the West, we are asking the question: why are humans unhappy?

The answer is simple. We have created a fast-lane society, though we do not have a cozy home and, without a cozy home, we do not have a mental state of nerve-relaxed personality. Without having a mental state of nerve-relaxed personality, we cannot face this fastness of the outer world; it's impossible.

Knowing this, we learn of our capabilities to control our inside. We are designed to manage stability in our hearts and minds and this will withstand as well as understand, our strong mental states. Would you chose to be a victim of life or become a wizard or warrior? The warrior poses in asana practice help us build strength and stability. Where are you when your feel strongest?

softly, slowly, calmly flows
a river of peace within

Day 236
Training Practice

How do we work with strong emotions when they arise?

The first thing to do is consciously note them.

When we note the emotions—the breath and sounds as emotions arise—we are training the mind. When difficult circumstances arise, we can default to the breathing that promotes calm.

When great pressure arises, you don't rise to the challenge, you fall to your level of training.

it is within the practice, and because of the practice, we transcend

Day 237
Embraced Emotion

Stay in the moment when difficulties and disappointment arrive. Learn from them because to do so is to learn about yourself.

Don't deny those moments. Don't push them away. Instead, engage in this kind of inner dialogue: *Ah, this is disappointment. Where is it resonating in my body? Where do I feel it? What does it feel like?*

When you are open to a stronger emotion like disappointment you can then let it pass through you. It is then a natural occurence, not avoided. Without denial, your life's journey can continue, rather than be detoured or stalled by pain.

embrace every experience
hold onto your heart

Day 238
Cognitive Ability

Just like the body heals on its own when it's wounded, so can the mind because it is designed with cognitive ability.

Your mind has limitless power to compensate for, and overpower, the loss of external stimulus. You are not only braver and stronger than you think, you are braver and stronger *because* you think and because of the ways you think: positively, calmly, meditatively, kindly, gracefully, thankfully.

we align with the universe when calm,
kind, positive, and thankful

Day 239
Discard

What world do you want? If it's not the one you see, then it's time to change, time to let go, maybe time to give up what you think you love best. Do not stay who you are to avoid who you can become.

What can you sacrifice as you feel drawn to the mystery of what's to come for you?

you are worthy of growth

Day 240
Hallelujah

We worry we are not enough, and that we are inadequate. Our own shadow terrifies us. We want the light on all the time. We embrace this imposter syndrome: "Oh, no, I'm not that great. It was nothing. I'm not really that innovative." We deny ourselves enlightenment because we stay in the shadows, with a forty-watt bulb turned on.

Turn around, open the window, let the sun in, beam with it. You are a glory maker, a shaker-up of souls, a shouter from the rooftops, a living hallelujah. Do not be afraid of being. Innovation, creativity, talent is our nature. Pair your purpose with goodness and celebrate. When you figure out how to let all the light in, you can show others how. Lead the parade; lift others and cheer them on.

our light shines brighter
when lighting another

Day 241
In Still

Silence is neither weak nor empty. It is a gift you can give yourself. It is priceless. The calm found through silence is profound. The ideas that spring forth after silence are infinite.

silence is a tool for peace and
creates space to hear the universe speak

Day 242
Alleviating Stress

When we experience a racing heart, and tense muscles, and sweaty palms, we can be assured we are dealing with stress.

Have you experienced these? Do you have other symptoms from stress?

These feelings are life energy flowing through your body, and you can redirect them to calm.

Yoga will make the reset easier and even seamless. As you practice yoga, the stress symptoms will hardly appear before you have engaged your superpower of peace.

center is balance, balance is calm,
calm is a superpower

Day 243
Imagine

Imagine…

The lyrics of John Lennon's song say it all. Take a few minutes to revisit the song.

Or simply think about this: what if we viewed the entire world population as our family?

It's amazing, isn't it? Suddenly, the circle expands. We feel for every person. We want to help others. Every living creature and every life-form together in peace and harmony.

We can never love and care too much when our intentions are pure.

imagine a world of peace,
no separation, borders, materialism

Day 244
Expansion

When we turn our attention to something, energy naturally begins to shift. Where our focus goes, energy flows. When we maintain that attention, even when discomfort or difficulties arise, then change is even more profound. What we focus on expands.

Keep track of where you direct your energy—keep a check on it.

energy is moving,
be aware of its direction

Day 245
Now

Creativity happens when we focus on the here and now. Innovation takes place when we concentrate on the moment and trust the ideas we hear in the silence. Life happens in each moment.

create, co-create, conspire
for goodness now

Day 246
Dream Another Dream

What is one thing you have now that you once dreamed of?

Likely you focused because you wanted it so much.

Focus feeds a river of energy. Have you learned from some of the challenges on your way to the dream come true?

When we learn from our challenges in attaining a dream, we can use the lesson learned in reaching another goal. That is, if we dare to dream another dream.

Now, dream another dream today and, as you move through your day, add details to your new dream, as many details as you can.

dream now, dream always, dream big

Day 247
Rise of the Goddess

Life is not only about what happens in our lives; it's about who we choose to be when we're in the space of what happens. Our approach determines whether we will create miracles. Yoga is not just getting into a pose, it's who you are on the way into the pose.

The world is full of miracles when we are receptive to seeing them. It can be our mission to create them also.

Ask yourself: "Who would you have me meet, and who can I serve?"

celebrate your light and fall in love
with your magnificent possibilities

Day 248
Challenge Is the Way

Many view difficult times as a challenge, often unbearable.

Consider a different viewpoint: difficult times allow for motivational challenge. Challenges can inspire us to place a higher value on our spiritual life. Conflict and obstacles are destined to be on the path.

In difficulty, we think, rest, develop, innovate, create, and learn.

Traveling the path of a challenge is the journey to being our own hero.

Are you avoiding pain? How brave are you?

pain will come; use it to define
and redesign a great you

Day 249
Here

Simplify, simplify. Create something from nothing, go for a walk, or write in a journal. One small step in the direction of your goals moves you with the path of here.

Affirm for yourself: I am already here.

your presence is your journey

Samadhi: The 8th Limb

The eighth limb of yoga, samadhi, is the culmination of practice and the beginning of a new journey only experienced by being moved by the previous seven limbs, then allowing the eighth to arrive and be. It cannot be chased, netted, or trapped. The deepest state of mental concentration simply arrives.

Samadhi cannot be explained to its fullest in words. It cannot be demonstrated in an action. It has to be experienced to understand its enlightenment, peace, bliss, ecstasy, love, and interconnected nature of reality.

Samadhi means "integration." It becomes a responsibility to integrate and live from this wisdom, in places we visit and in our relationships. Yoga never ends. We never get to a destination. Our gift is our presence, to be intimate with what is happening now in our lives just as they are and not how we think they should be.

I chose to include the most days of reflection in the samadhi section because it is the beginning of waking up to what is around us. Without living from this wisdom of our connected nature, no matter how great the awakening, our old habits we will likely take us back at the first yama.

We are all subject to the cultures we live in and, with awareness of our interconnectedness, we aim to get along with others; we are always in relationship.

We practice our ethics and limbs to match our situations and relationships. Embodying the yamas as our ethical framework offers light to respond to ever-changing situations with understanding, kindness, and compassion. Responding this way is a return to authenticity. It is an awakening from a self-centred reality and supports us to contribute harmony to others. It facilitates a greater existential reality of life and death. Responding by the principles of nonviolence, honesty, non-stealing, using energy wisely, and not accumulating more than we need, we align more closely and authentically with others and our heart.

The Samadhi Days

Day 250
Your Place, Your Space

Yoga studios are in commercial centres or homes, in parks or parking lots, and on beaches. They are anywhere yoga instruction takes place. Simple or complex, heated or humidified, they all have one thing in common: sanctuary.

Can you make one room or space in your home a sacred space for you and yoga?

If you do this, it becomes a part of your ritual and a reminder of the beauty in life and in you.

it is healthy to create a space
reflecting our sacred beauty

Day 251
Cultivate Benevolence

Once we have cultivated and felt deep union, peace, and love within our own heart, we are able to share and genuinely give to others. Metta prayer is one type of meditation practice designed to open the heart and share this loving kind attitude with others.

May we be happy and may we be healthy.

May we ride the waves of our lives.

May we live in peace.

cultivate a loving kindness attitude
towards ourselves and others

Day 252
Dance

Loneliness aches for a compass.

The body, mind, and soul seek a guide through the mountains of life. The ego calls out for reference points that stroke the loneliness.

Enlightenment says, "Go right, go left, take a step into the infinite. Hand over heart, feel the rhythm, onward in love."

How do you dance between loneliness and enlightenment?

choose love as your dance partner
and keep on dancing

Day 253
Karma

You are an essential element of an interconnected web of wholeness.

Within that web is the Buddhist idea of karma—the belief that every action we take has an effect. It's been said, until you understand karma, nothing is going to change.

Karma also enhances ethics; they are intimate.

Buddhism explains this simply: bad seeds=bad fruit… good seeds, good fruit. For Buddhists, karma explains inequality. Karma's concept reminds people to take responsibility for their actions.

Can you expand your realization to include how important your role and responsibility is?

your life is your karma—
your actions can transform humanity

Day 254
Women's Strength

Women's empowerment encompasses a range of processes that serve as the building of confidence, so a person feels supported and strong enough within themself to make transformational choices, then continue toward further action and achieve results.

Through the process, an individual becomes an agent of change. Simply put: it's the can-do factor.

How do we empower girls and women?

You change the world.

with empowerment we step into
"I can and I will"

Day 255
Gaining Wisdom

When we explore the concept of impermanence—which is central to Buddhist practice—we begin to gain wisdom. In learning how we respond to what comes and goes we then become masterful at understanding the concept of coming and going, of letting go, of widening the gaps between events, of responding in love.

joy and wisdom embody
the peaceable person

Day 256
Life Energy

When we begin to embody the world through the eyes, fingertips, nose, ears, and heart-feelings of yoga, then the land is the land, everything vibrates, everything is energy. There is ground, there are hills and rivers. With wisdom we learn every-thing is life and we are life.

we are nature, everything
and everyone is energy

Day 251
Pleasure Seekers

Humans crave happiness. Humans want to avoid suffering. We deny the reality of suffering and work so hard to make this happen. We chase happiness fiercely as though with a butterfly net through a grove where there are no butterflies. We avoid pain and therefore fall out of touch with happiness.

no net is required to capture
the nuances of life—only an open heart

Day 258
Open Intentions

When I am open to all possibilities, in a natural, unforced way, without the intent of chasing, then I can be freely curious, forever the explorer, and sit at my campfire at night in awe of the wonders of the world.

every day is a masterclass
every answer is love

Day 259
Adventure

A sacred contract with peace creates a journey of adventure, guarantees uncertainty, requires a faithful courage in the bigger picture of energy.

When we trust in process, we journey through fun times, mutually beneficial relationships, and encounter pleasant experiences. Adventurous peaceful attitudes continue to follow bliss.

be curious, be open,
be purely and beautifully you

Day 260
Friend Space

As social beings for whom sharing is life-affirming, we need loving friendships. With this truth for all, then it is only natural that our friends will have friends that are not just us. This is true sharing of and with each other. This creates a tribe, and the stronger the tribe, the stronger and more independent we feel, causing less drama, dependency, and jealousy.

Notice the freedom from grasping and self-doubt. Notice the power of knowing who you are is no longer dependent on someone else's actions.

more freedom
deeper friendships

Day 261
Haven

We are each capable of achieving more than we ever imagined. Love is the way. It's important to have a place to centre yourself, a place to be yourself, a place to trust and call home. Some secure safe haven. A place that is yours to grow, enjoy, to play in, to be you with all things you love. We need a haven to just be.

surround yourself with what you love

Day 262
I Am Enough

Sometimes you need a reminder you are enough right now, without exception. If you have trouble believing that, make a list of all the things you love and value about yourself.

Each night, write one thing you love and value about yourself. Once your list is started, sit in your meditation with the mantra "I am enough." Repeat the words as you inhale and exhale.

every body and every spirit
are more than enough

Day 263
Dimmer Switch

We know that when we turn the dial of a dimmer switch, the light fades and eventually we are in darkness. When we turn it the other way, the room gradually becomes lighter and reaches the maximum potential of whatever bulb is installed.

What about life? Is that ethereal dial limitless? How light can it be? How bright can it be? Is light infinite in its property to rise like a sun inside us and shine on and for the world?

we are light makers and light givers

Day 264
Understanding Mantra

Man means mind and *tra* signifies transport or vehicle (a delivery system). A mantra is an instrument of the mind—a powerful sound or vibration that is transported by and through your mind and body. Your mind does not repeat positives naturally, which is why repeating positive mantras is essential for well-being.

mantra vibrations bring harmony
to mind, body, and soul

Day 265
Easy Peasy

Mantras are meant to bring us back to simplicity. They guide us out of the details of a complex world.

When we return to simplicity, we touch happiness, hold joy, and dance in the peace of it all. Use mantra as a tool to further develop your own meditation or yoga practice by speaking to yourself through mantra as often as you can.

use a mantra to keep the mind focused
and the body dancing

Day 266
Openness

When our hearts are open, every person and thing, no matter their role in life, can provide a lesson. Openness allows us to receive. The world does not change, we change.

we are all learning
we are all teaching

Day 267
Truthful, Neighbourly

We move to a new home and do not know the neighbours. Or someone moves in next door in our community. Which way do we lean? Fear or love? It is natural— a human condition based on surviving—to go to fear. However the way forward is to recognize fear, then pour forth love. That is the way of the heart.

we more than need each other,
we are each other

Day 268
Attachment and Caring

Attachment is to cry over the broken plate that meant a lot to you, and to be angry with the person who dropped it. Caring is to see the pain in the accident-maker's eyes and for them to mean more to you than the plate.

Creativity is to take the broken pieces and make something greater than the plate. That can be a ceremony of ceramic dust returning to the earth, it can be two tiny plates glued and shaped then shared, one for you and one for the person who broke it. It can be the activity of sharing the after effects, or it can be the surprise when the activity has been done alone.

Attachment is akin to possession. Caring is closer to forgiveness.

I choose caring. I choose to forgive.

to cling to an object or person is
to limit your freedom and restrict theirs

Day 269
Empty Knapsack

Looking back over your life, how many weeks, months, even years, have you wasted anguishing over something you didn't get from a parent, a spouse, or from life?

Did all of that anguish serve you? Or would it have been more skillful to have received fully the experience of the loss, accepted it as it was, and then to have allowed your emotions to go on to experience what was possible in each present moment?

More importantly, are you still caught in an endless cycle of a wanting mind, imagining the next accomplishment, change in relationship, or piece of recognition that will make you happy?

Let go of the suitcase filled with dozens of sorrys, stacked with loss, bursting with anger—so full that you had to sit on it to zip it up. When will the suitcase explode? Has it imploded enough?

Pause now, dear soul, and visualise leaving the suitcase on the luggage carousel. Let it sit in lost and found. Your life is here. Your life happens here, now, in this moment. Grab an empty knapsack. Put only goodness in it.

release the heavy loads.
now, bask in your spectacular beauty

Day 270
Powerful Self-Speech

It is okay to want the best for myself and to pursue the things that bring me joy and happiness. I can choose positive thoughts. I understand the power of my self-talk and choose to select thoughts that are uplifting and empowering. I let my happiness be visible to others. My happiness overflows from me. I can use my happiness to bring joy to others. I am strong. I have many strengths to navigate the ups and downs of my life. I am tougher and braver than I look. I am becoming. I am becoming the person I want to be. Each day, I act to make myself more the person I aspire to be. My life is moving forward perfectly. Each bump in the road is there for a reason. Everything is happening according to a greater plan. I am confident in my decisions. I am creator of my own destiny. I stand behind the things I do and say. I surround myself with loving people. I choose the people I allow into my life. I surround myself with people who love and adore me.

the words we choose
are the highest form of respect
we give ourselves

Day 271
You Are Love

Within your relationship with another are specific lessons. Perhaps you are growing through group work or working together—like in school when asked to get a partner or pair up to create a play, a picture, or a report. In those cases, we learned about the other person's style. In those collaborations, did we look at our own style? In the grown-up version, we get to be more insightful analysts.

In our partnerships, we can expand each other's horizons, discover another type of humour, laugh more, celebrate more, hug more.

In meeting the person you believe you can spend the rest of your life with, you can understand this means changing together, ebbing, and flowing, respecting each other's space and habits. This is to grow in a partnership of kindness and peacefulness.

Your greatest love story of all time is your relationship with yourself. How you measure your relationship with anyone else is a direct reflection of how you relate to yourself. If you're looking to find the love of your life, look no further: you are that love.

we are relationship architects coordinating
with designers
who mirror our love

Day 272
Lights Fade

It seems to be something humans do: get fearful when the sunlight slips away and physical darkness moves in. We are so used to light fixtures and flipping on a switch that we have become strangers to navigating our way in the dark… and we have confused the dark with the unknown. When we accept that, no matter the ambiance, we are all-knowing creatures, then we can move comfortably without fear in our physical and emotional world.

clarity of thought thrives
with the lights out, for it is in the dark
when we are most ourselves

Day 273
Darkness

There are times when we need to sit in the shadows, to lie at the bottom of the dry well in the darkness. Creating darkness, in order to think (like turning off a computer, a lamp, or a phone), can transport us to a kingdom where we can be alone and think about the value of being in the dark. When we immerse ourselves in the silence of all the darkness, one could say we are darkness-ing: absorbing the lessons dark has to offer.

Being creative in and with the dark can help train us for the difficulties that are inevitable. Becoming familiar with the physical dark can be a kind of resilience training, and allow us to appreciate the dark as we do the light.

darkness offers many gifts
for us to shine in the light

Day 274
Deep Generosity

When we let go, we find ourselves in deep generosity. When we give of our talents and skills or our possessions in generous measures, we open ourselves to freedom. In giving, we liberate ourselves.

remain empty to be full—
we are enough and there is always enough

Day 275
Practice Makes Ritual

When we participate in consistent goodness, to others and to ourselves, we create a lifetime pattern of love. Simple things like giving gratitude for having a cup from which to drink—and imagining all the people who made the cup, glazed the cup, transported the cup, sold the cup—brings with it so much more meaning to the sip you take. That cup of tea becomes ceremonial, honoring all those who are part of it.

the opportunity to celebrate
is everywhere in everything

Day 276
It All Has to Mean Something

We have these four letters, L-I-F-E, and they pack so much power. We say it and, literally, we hold our life in our hands. Sometimes another holds our life in their hands. How can such a small word, a combo of four letters, mean so much and yet be indefinable? It is kind of like the ocean with currents going one way or another, with high tides, and low tides, so deep in places that the sun cannot reach such depths… yet still there are lifeforms.

It all means something… yoga brings us closer to understanding our love story, the story we call life.

keep falling in love—every moment
is a new chance to fall

Day 277
Love

Meaningful moments are private ones of peace, grace, and connection. They create meaningful smiles from ecstasy meeting rapture—leading to our heart overflowing with joy.

Each of us has our own path, divinely created. We learn to trust more, to celebrate ourselves, and to fall in love with the infinite possibilities all within the open source of uncertainty. Love is bliss.

we are each a blissful, divine,
loving piece of creation

Day 278
You Are Sky

Karma is like the ocean bird that lands and takes off, flies for days above oceans, or perches on a railing right outside your window and squawks nonstop. Karma wakes you with song or siren and bids you goodnight with sweet dreams or nightmares. It is ever present; it creates you; you create it. Yet, when we close the gap with goodness, gain the skills to peace, and rise, we can glide in the clear sky with those same winged miracles, tipping our wings to compassion and love.

every moment matters—we can fly

Day 279
Compassionate Core

Our motivation to do good comes from our core values, which change over time based on our experiences. Yoga brings a buffet of healthy choices for us to select from. When we taste the nectar of compassion, we understand we have known no equal. Then the quest begins to cultivate and to expand compassion. We commit to a journey to the centre of our loving selves—beyond emotional responses—to a place where real compassion resides.

when compassion prevails,
our behavior is loving and kind

Day 280
Application

To thoroughly enjoy the freedom of the eight limbs of yoga, one will practice being—not chase being, not covet being, simply practice being by being still. The aim is being over doing, and feeling over forcing.

One can create scenarios to practice that can build a kind of muscle memory of how to simply be.

Keep practicing how to be the most graceful being you are. That is the work of a hero.

the best practice is real life
and life is happening for you

Day 281
Benefiting from the Results

Remember the Third Moment (days 165-170) can be easy to miss. Aim your focus and awareness on the moment before you connect emotion and thought. Aim not to let them connect or solidify. Instead, aim to observe the emotion for what it is. You can find the Third Moment in the instant between reading a hurtful email and shooting back a nasty reply. It is between seeing your favourite tasty treat and reaching for it. It is in these spaces, these instants between the moments, you can practice the Third Moment Method.

emotions are not reality—
we can interact more pleasantly
with ourselves and others

Day 282
Looks Can Be Deceiving

Do not mistake a slower response for a lack of enthusiasm. A well-practiced sage knows when to act and when to let things go. In time, we can all develop that skill. Every situation has an energy, a vibration—an energetic statement—and every response, even no response, is a reply to that energy.

we are master of our moments

Day 283
Three Stages to Depth

We apply effort, then we are met with resistance. We let go and we surrender. These are the stages we go through when we are breaking out of limitation, moving to be more open to the superpower that is life and love.

we get where we are going
and we are exactly where we need to be

Day 284
A Tangled Structure

It is when we give up, in the letting-go way, and abandon (not sweep under the carpet) the twisted mess we've created from a perceived problem that we find clarity… to approach the situation from another angle or witness it has unfurled without our help. This is especially true of emotional trauma.

there is a soul solution to all
perceived problems because all problems
are perception

Day 285
Epiphanies

Epiphanies seem to arrive from nowhere. Perhaps that nowhere is a sacred space beyond our limits and the epiphany is a gift for us doing our soul work and is greatness opening up inside us. A light for us from a brighter and more peaceful place than we could ever imagine.

There is wonder, ease, and grace following epiphany. One can feel proud of this wondrous power emerging from within and question if it came from some other realm. It is then we can embrace those realms within us. It is only then we approach coherence and begin to be powerfully present. To be natural and light and feel that we are surfers riding waves in the great ocean of existence.

energy and flow is deeper when we let go

Day 286
Waterway

Buddhism compares life to a river. We can all picture ourselves flowing downstream or fighting upstream. We get the picture in our minds right away... a river... each of ours a unique waterway with or without surrounding scenery, some carrying solids, dissolved or whole.

   As the water in the river is never the same in one spot, neither is life each day the same as the previous, even though it might, on the surface, look that way. Where we get stuck in our relationships, jobs, thinking, or ideas, we can apply this image and trust letting go of the shore, the branch, the thought, the person, or holding onto the rock we think we need.

holding on is slow and letting go we flow

Day 287
Endurance

The more we go after being comfortable, the more cautious we become, and the less we risk and adventure. At some point, comfort becomes so important that we are unable to take any hardship if it comes along—and it always does because life is contrast. To live fully is to appreciate comfort, to recognize hardship, and to be able to float between the two with little drama and much fluidity.

endurance is maintaining
intensity and balance

Day 288
Gift Within Hardship

Westerners are said to suffer from the disease of preciousness, meaning we have little ability or willingness to put up with discomfort. This hinders our spiritual development.

Change produces discomfort and, in turning away from hardship, we walk away from change. The thing is—when we walk away from change, we discount opportunity and we say no to growth. Change actually happens *for* us and not *to* us.

Can you begin to see each challenge as the path to choose for growth?

when change crashes into us
we can handle great things

Day 289
Creativity

Imagination is a prerequisite for the spiritual life. Without it we would not be able to visualize ourselves in a changed mode.

We need to be able to imagine ourselves as changed. We need to know change so we can empathize and sympathize with others.

compassion leaves an imprint
on the heart—ours and others

Day 290
Capability

We daydream, fantasize, story-tell, fall in love, save money, exaggerate. All these require imagination. To consciously use our imagination in order to develop a greater empathy with others is not as common, yet it is what we need to do to progress spiritually.

How does imagination serve you in your life?

imagination means our capacity
for love is infinite

Day 291
Empathy

When we understand someone else's suffering we are presenting them with an incredible gift of love.

When we cannot understand the suffering of another, then we cannot fully know love.

deep self-love is
the uniting love of the universe

Day 292
Forgive Often

Forgiveness is a superpower. The qualities that contribute to being a truthful forgiver are courage and integrity. Where people get mixed up is in thinking by forgiving, they are ignoring the truth of suffering. This is not the case. Forgiveness is peacemaking and peace giving. It does not erase any truth; it brings light to it.

forgiveness brings light

Day 293
True Love

True love is for the mastercrafters of loving lives; we are all serving an apprenticeship to an unseen master who is constantly teaching us love, to give grace, forgiveness, compassion, and a thousand other bright stars of value.

the quest for truth is the journey to love

Day 294
No Expiry

Forgiveness has no shelf life. It can be brought down from the shelf and applied—offered—at any time. It can also be requested, as in, "Can you forgive me?" Forgiveness is an ongoing form of love, it affirms our respect for others and for ourselves. Writing a forgiveness list is a powerful process. Write your forgiveness list now.

forgiveness is freedom and peace

Day 295
Sorry from the Heart

There is no meaning in the word sorry unless there is emotion behind it. First must come responsibility… we have to admit our error, take ourselves to the mirror, and say, "Yes, I did this. I made a terrible mistake." Only then can forgiveness be requested and/or given to ourself or to another human.

An apology functions this way reciprocally. A sorry delivered to us in words without emotion—from another—is meaningless to them and does not help their growth—if it is not delivered with authenticity.

sorry is made up of more than words

Day 296
Rise and Shine

Owning our greatness is not selfish: rather it is essential if we want to help others. We help no one by playing small. Not ourselves. Not others. If we are not aligning our authentic greatness with our actions, then what are we doing?

our biggest fear is not that we are small,
it is that we are actually larger than life

Day 297
Authentic Apology

When we genuinely apologize, we are entering a path of humility. We are healing our soul. We are loving towards ourselves and others. There is a vibrational shift in our actions to not repeat the automatic pattern of that mistake anymore. We genuinely step towards a better version of ourselves.

we have the power to heal and transform

Day 298
After Sorry

We will never know the weight of a wrong, until we apologize and feel that burden lift. It is a shakiness that weakens us when it is lifted. Ideally, we'd never do anything that would require an apology, however, we are human and imperfectly perfect. Breathing is a safe place of return after delivering an apology, or after forgiving the self or another. We need space to allow the after-effect of the emotion and statement to become another kind of energy. Give yourself conditions to relax within, and lots of space. Be gentle with yourself through this process.

positive or negative or resolving
emotional statements create
physical symptoms we can nurture

Day 299
Partnerships

We thrive in partnerships. We thrive when we admit we are still learning. We succeed in relationships when we talk it out and truly listen to the other person.

Great partners stand together and move in harmony. They support each other's journey and know it is necessary to have space. Their consideration of one another lends itself to the kind of thoughtfulness where, when the lights are off in the bedroom and one wants to read, a booklight is accessed. That kind of consideration doesn't overpower the partner, yet it finds a healthy balance of energy.

we're here for a human experience;
relationship is yoga

Day 300
All We Need Is Love

We need to love ourselves first. Otherwise, we may feel suffocated in a relationship. We cannot express love unconditionally when we are hung up in confusion over how we feel and are not intimate with ourselves.

love yourself first and then
you can truly love another

Day 301
Into Love

As with anything you consider important, you can learn to just show up and hope for the best. You want to plan well. Evaluate clearly. Play the odds. In no way am I suggesting this is simple. It takes tremendous presence and super-human commitment to walk into this fire.

Instead of flinging yourself kamikaze-like into the flame of love, you can train to work in the heat.

commit to full, present participation—
you are born to handle life's beautiful fire

Day 302
Love Is Everywhere

At the point where love is the landscape, we have succeeded in immersing ourselves in it, we have cultivated community, and we can commune with others. The way to all loving ways is love. Is that an oversimplification? Not when you understand love is life, peace, grace, values, compassion, and a thousand more qualities.

the path of love is open to all

Day 303
All You Seek Is Within

If a person has not experienced self-love, there is no chance that person can love another, even though it is love they require to grow. A person cannot give what they do not have. A person cannot change what is not present. With guidance a person can seemingly make something out of nothing because we are all energy, and we naturally gravitate to the next best feeling, then the next best step, discovering the path to self-love.

love is our essence—
every human has the potential
for cultivating love

Day 304
Friends First

In companionship and caring we experience friendship and camaraderie. We find joy in our own hearts as we bring it out in the hearts of another—and they bring it out in us. Then, through this progression of friendship, of tribe, of trust, of back-and-forth discovery, love sparks and we move to love. That is a healthy development.

love and life are processes

Day 305
Rise in Love

There is no descent or decline into love, only an arising. When love grows it brings the whole garden of life into an illuminating bloom. Even in the darkest times, true love thrives. This has been proven over again during times of war when families were separated.

love is a climbing rose on the arbour of life

Day 306
Back and Forth

Like a pendulum, every one of us swings back and forth between needing independence and togetherness. Go far in the direction of independence and it is time to swing back toward togetherness. This happens for all of us.

there is a natural rhythm to life

Day 307
Faith

The principle of any faith-based practice is a good heart.

The paths the heart can take are many, and they are all in the community of service. The more we serve, the stronger our hearts. The kinder we are, the stronger the beat. The core being of who you are, of who we all are, is goodness.

Say: "I am good. All beings possess goodness."

start with the good heart
expand to the smart heart

Day 308
Beyond Barriers

When your love for each other is greater than your need for each other then you are in a pleasant relationship. Strive to understand the barriers which are thrown up in front of you—like grasping or lack. Barriers are also impermanent and can shift to your advantage as you give attention to them. Letting go is also letting love.

healthy relationships contribute to
rather than contaminate our lives

Day 309
Compassion Foundation

When compassion is on a solid foundation, then no matter the behaviour of another—no matter how negative—your capacity for compassion will not change. Compassion is compassion through and through. There are no grey areas.

encourage with words, act kindly,
and feel deeply while others experience
the ups and downs of life

Day 310
Deep Presence

True compassion cannot be shaken. It will never collapse. It is a form of love so great it is a vast mountain range of expression so wide and long it wraps around the entire world. Compassion flows from us when we relax judgment, heal trauma, listen generously, or bring groceries to someone in need. Ultimate compassion is our presence.

rooted in compassion is love
living compassion alleviates suffering

Day 311
Yoga Teacher

As a yoga teacher, it does not matter how many people come to my class. What matters is that my students walk in and feel peace and walk away feeling light and love. This means I am in constant process of growth, devotion, learning, embodying yoga. I prepare daily to customize teachings to help students return to themselves. Teaching yoga is humbling and profound. I am a yoga teacher and I will never stop being a student.

yoga is bigger than any ideas about yoga
yoga is more than you think it is
yoga never ends

Day 312
Breath Matters

What matters in my practice is the union of my breath with my movements and mind. There is no competition in me or with others. Yoga does not require anyone to do the longest headstand.

Nor is there a race to see who gets to nirvana first.

It does not matter how much I weigh, or the shape of my belly or thighs, or the thickness or thinness of my ankles. What is important is I am healthy and adventurous.

Can you be mindful of your movements as you transition pose to pose?

you are vitality and individuality
in mind, body, and soul

Day 313
No Opposites

Buddhism teaches us there are eight worldly concerns: gain and loss, praise and blame, pleasure and pain, happiness and unhappiness. Each is said to arrive with its twin—its opposite. Our mind processes this information into opposites.

For today let us remember yin and yang. They are two interlocked fish and neither exists without the other. Opposites can appear completely different, though we can see them now as an expansion, something alive between them and not on a course for collision, no separation. In relation they evolve. The differences are the unity.

difference and unity are inseparable;
though we look different, we are one

Day 314
Wouldn't II Be Nice...

Really, wouldn't it be great if life went from one happy event to another? Where there was no personal hell? Buddhists would laugh at us for wanting this—albeit in a nice, joking, non-judging way. When will we learn we are supposed to go through times of pain and feelings of loss and confusion—and that growth comes when we learn to go through them and reduce their severity by finding something in them to be grateful for, or understanding how permanently we are perceiving them? The only way out is to go through.

pain is a vital element of love.
pain and love create a foundation of
our infinite power

Day 315
Storytelling

We are experts at making loss into a dramatic novella rather than accepting it as a normal part of life. When we create stories about these events, we make ourselves a character, which creates a false identity. In this way, we move away from our true heart and soul. By creating the story, and retelling it, we entrench ourselves further into the false identity.

We don't have to be story-makers in the dramatic category. We can create a statement of passage to frame the event and create a going-forward story narrating the greatness from an event which is hardly memorable since the greatness has far surpassed the pain. Our storytelling skills can create comedies, thrillers, and love stories.

What kind of story will you express to the world?

we can inspire, heal, connect deeply, and understand others through story-telling

Day 316
Movement as Medicine

There's a pond in the woods that sort of sits there, stagnating. There is no spring that feeds it, only the annual rainfall keeps it within a range of pond-ness. There is so little about it that changes… it just sits. Sure, it sustains some life and serves a purpose, yet it is without the action a lively stream, a babbling brook, a raging river, or an active lake possesses. At best it has a foot of murky water, at worst it is mud.

It is the same for happiness. I know, wait, that's not a mistake. We can stagnate in one state. If we are perpetually on the same level of happiness, that is not dynamic and energetic and evolving. It's sort of muddy. In that state of "just happy," we atrophy. We lose our focus. We need a steady supply of fresh water in the way of lessons to keep us growing and moving upstream to other versions of happy, and sad, and elation, and sorrow, and devastation, perhaps enlightenment. Fortunately, we are not stuck out in the woods. We have arms and legs and minds and can choose to immerse ourselves in all kinds of activities, relationships, personal development, and events.

the difference between
medicine and poison is dose

Day 317
One Love

No matter how much chanting we do, or how many poses we hold, or how many breaths we control, or even how deep we go in meditation, the most important light we can ignite is the light of love. Sages have called yoga a spark: once lit, it never extinguishes.

we are here to grow in and through love

Day 318
Every Moment Matters

There is no situation from which you cannot emerge wiser, stronger, and more determined to create success. Don't ask what meaning your life has; ask what meaning will you make of it.

Einstein, when asked to define time, said, "Illusion."

Any story you tell that includes *I wish I had time*, know the time is now. Mail the card, write to a person, express what you want to say to others. If you do not, the not doing will continue to be a part of your journey.

You don't have to carry anything that brings you down; you can rewrite any script to make it beautiful and healed and holy for you. Everything is energy.

let love be our intention for every word,
movement, and moment; this is how
we can leave the world a better place
than we found it

Day 319
Feed the Possibility

To be a teacher, rise to the calling. It's easy to be seduced by negativity; our reactivity is hungry. Starve the problems to rise above yourself. When we do that, everything outside serving becomes minor. What then becomes major are the new skills, people, places, and events we'll need to teach.

rising is taking action towards
the direction you want to go—
the universe will meet you

Day 320
Spark Love

Teachers become teachers through the depths of experiences. Without experience one can only parrot what someone else says without thinking or understanding.

There's a difference between a wise teacher and one who parrots. The latter mimics and repeats. There's never an experience giving depth to anything they speak about.

Teachers who teach from the heart trust their students; their compelling lessons arrive at a vibrational level so that they can meet the students where the students are.

My goal as a teacher is to add oxygen to the fire of learning, to spark the embers of love burning in each student's heart, and to rekindle the fire when the joyful flame goes out of life.

teaching is sacred; life is sacred

Day 321
Planting Seeds

I am grateful beyond words to be a yoga teacher. Simultaneously, I act according to understanding I will never stop being a student. I am an eternal seeker of ancient wisdom the great minds have left for us, to ease our hearts, and to love. In lieu of teaching what you know, teach what the student does not know.

teaching yoga is a conversation
and an intimate dance

Day 322
As Above, So Below

The sun and moon cast their light on the world regardless of the way others feel about them. The sun and moon are loved, admired, studied, neglected, unseen by some, yet they maintain their strength and power. Like the sun and moon, you are a part of a powerful interconnection.

we are sun and moon
we are love, strength, and beauty

Day 323
Let Go

We practice flow in yoga so as to not get stuck. We inhale, exhale, and keep moving. We do not stay with the inhale or exhale; we practice letting it go. Over and over again we let the breath go. Over and over, we let the poses go.

How many times should each pose be repeated? Until we learn to let go with ease and gratitude, until we feel inner confidence, until we trust in the process which informs us we are safe and that letting go is okay.

there's nothing to let go of because
there's nothing to hold onto—
letting go is letting love

Day 324
I love Me

When you forget about the idea of people loving you before you love yourself, then you can focus less on what's happening outside you and around you, and turn inward to discover your truth and fall in love with magnificent you.

turn the light of love within;
capture and romance your own heart

Day 325
Everyone Is Okay

We change our clothes when they are worn out, or when we find them impractical, or even when our tastes change and we want to embrace a different brand—perhaps a higher quality or an ethical manufacturer. We can do the same with people. If you are drained from those around you, then it's time to change it up. Shake up your social circle. This benevolent, self-love requires courage. Imagine you're being cued to be magnanimous to yourself for your future—and for the world.

Who are you not to be your best?

friends are forever in the heart—
be not afraid of a brand new start

Day 326
Interbeing

When we're in relationships, our views of ourselves change. The opinions of others have a profound impact on what we believe about ourselves. Through this we can lose sight of our goals and someone else's goals can appear as our own… and we might be surprised and ask, when did that happen?

Some intertwining is normal, as is collaboration, and resetting joint goals. When we open to another, through intimacy, we are influenced by their values and dreams, and they are affected by ours. Being aware of this is a positive attribute. The awareness of this intertwining can improve the quality and longevity of our relationships.

independence and collaboration
are a great team

Day 327
Recovery

A breakup is an ending, not a rejection. It might not feel like that initially, yet it's an important thing to remember. When your heart has been broken, it can take a while to find your way back to whole. You will return. Healing from a broken heart is as much a physical process as an emotional one. It's similar to recovering from an addiction, which is why it feels so hard and is so painful.

People change, and when it's the person we love who has changed it can feel breathtakingly painful. As hard as it is, don't take this personally. The relationship dance between the two of you has come to an end. In time you will find your strength and clarity around this, and you will be grateful for the wisdom that has come from the mess. In the meantime, how can you be gentle with yourself?

slow, steady, gentle. care for your heart first

Day 328
Truth and Dare

Truth and dare are a part of our journey as we move through life. They are equally opportune. When we dare to dream, we dare to aspire to a new level of consciousness. We can feel a little defeated when resistance shows up. That resistance is there to make us work hard to rise from where we are to where we want to be. This is part of the truth. The next part is to combine the truth and dare and understand that the strength is found within the possibility which, with strong ethics, becomes a probability… which, in the longer term, manifests as what you envisioned or shows up as something more profound.

What is one thing you can do today to stand in your truth?

dare to discover your authentic self.
be the truth of your heart and soul

Day 329
Tracking Your Growth

There may have been a doorway in your home growing up where someone marked your height, or a relative may have seen you once a year and commented on how you had grown—like a weed, they might have said. Those measurements are not accurate in the depth to which your roots have extended into the core of life. Or how much your soul has taken on in the passing years as you endured suffering, experienced abuse, and or celebrated milestones. Roots run deep; your roots are deep. If you look back, let it be only to see how far you have grown.

What could you notice today as a hell you survived? Can you see how important it is now?

growth is not linear—growth is nature
you are nature

Day 330
You Are More

We are not the sum of what we know from books and classrooms and videos. We are the sum of all we have known, all we will know, can know, could know. What I mean is if you stay in a secure pod, knowing only what you know and having only what you have, then it is impossible to go beyond, or see beyond. If you believe there are more roles for you to play, more dreams for you to dream, and more adventures for you to, well, adventure on! You are so much more than what you think you know.

open closed windows, invite the storm in,
run toward the sun, dance with the moon

Day 331
Confident Confidence

Walk in the rain, splash in the puddles, know there is a towel at home and, if you realize there isn't, then know you will improvise. That is optimism. A kind of confident optimism. A version of trust.

There is a difference between foolhardy and wonderstruck. When we are in awe of our environment, and can wait calmly in the storm, catching snowflakes on our tongue, harboring a drenched sparrow, reassuring a frightened child, and when we choose the time to put the sparrow under our coat, put the child on our shoulders, and march to the house a thousand miles away, then we are wise and confident.

the most dangerous storms are inside us—
within, we can create what's around us.
we are the managers
of our thoughts and emotions

Day 332
Cultivating Love

When we cultivate abilities to bring love into all aspects of our life and to all people we encounter, we are in a state of thriving. At that point, we are aware we have much more to learn, yet we know the learning will be a privilege and pleasure because of our understanding of the nature of life—of pain and joy, of the necessary ebb and flow. We will welcome it.

How can you cultivate a loving presence today?

love is like water:
we cannot live without it

Day 333
Tend to Thoughts

A mind filled with doubt is like an overgrown garden. It's overwhelming to begin cleaning up—how does one know where to start? Which are weeds? Weeds are a construct of someone's classification—maybe dandelions can be more useful than hydrangea.

What of these self-doubts? How are they stacked and scattered in you? Are there some which reside in your right foot, which stop you from taking that first step on a hike in the mountains or is that step connected to your fear of bears? Do you doubt you are prepared for the hike? Is that because you have not processed memories of a previous hike? Have you set the bar high and are ready to fail before you start? Would that be a failure—to re-evaluate the route?

Would a walk in the park be a cop-out? How can there be so much chatter in the moments it takes to tie a shoelace?

At some point, a review of the whole doubting self is necessary to restart the process of cultivating all the plants you want in your garden—all the thoughts you want in your head.

This can begin with making a list of your doubts. It unclutters the mind. It's the start of creating the rows and organizing the priorities and understanding the care needed for each doubt.

writing unburdens us and helps us focus on what matters most

Day 334
Practice Not Perfect

I believe my imperfections are what led me to teaching. Yoga classes I attended gave me technique and the ability to be in my body. I remember seeking out yoga classes when I thought I was falling apart, and I remember I practiced yoga just to stay together. Now, I know exactly who I am when I step on my mat.

When I discovered how life comes together through practice, when I knew yoga had healed my wounds, only then, fifteen years of yoga classes later, was I compelled to share with others. It is my way of service; teaching is my contribution to the world. May it be a better place than I found it.

As a teacher, I am always learning. Every moment is a new chance to fall in love; every breath is fresh.

a wise teacher is a student
endlessly falling in love

Day 335
Solvation

There is salvation and then a twist on redemption—I call it solvation. It refers to how we don't really solve things, we manage them. We might ask ourselves, am I here to solve a problem or here to solve my feelings about this problem?

Usually it is the latter, and it is productive. It means we can give the problem space, be free-thinking and open to a solution to the problem. There's great space and wisdom in that distinction. The space teaches that we are more than our feelings from which we can discern, organize, even rewrite our thoughts and emotions. Then we can expand to include awareness. From there we can create our own experience.

within us lives a kingdom of solutions

Day 336
Written Wounds

One powerful method which helps a person endure pain is to write out (on paper) the feelings associated with that pain. Whenever there's a hurricane of emotions inside you, let them out through a pen. Heartfelt stories will net serenity. Writing the wounds in the presence of your therapist—the journal—is highly cathartic.

love letters to ourselves are words of heart

Day 331
Non-Attachment

Everything that has a hold on us keeps us hostage and has to be released. Whether we conjure a caped avatar of ourselves, armed with weaponry that will combat the strongest emotional terrorist, or silently picture the melting of the ties that bind us to our pleasures, we have to move away from certain habits—and we know what they are—in order to advance to the life we dream about.

Release yourself from clinging. Embrace the unknown.

Breathe the air, enjoy weightlessness as you float freely down the river.

Leave the habits in your wake.

we are the hero of our own lives.
no one is coming for us

Day 338
Patterns

We are sometimes too much for someone, rather than not enough. We just don't realize that at the time because, when we're truly living life, we can't see it.

When we practice self-inquiry—turning our attention inward—and examine our sense of lack, we can see we were perhaps too much because of that sense of lack. Being too much may have overwhelmed the person we engaged with and, in their struggles with lack, became confused.

Presenting as too much out of a place of lack is not the same as presenting or knowing we are all more than enough.

Once we accept our value, we can dive into our insecurities and face the direction of self-worthiness. When we see the pattern, we can adjust and take another step into love, and another, over and over again.

What patterns do you recognize?

Can you feel a sense freedom from releasing feelings of dissatisfaction and lack?

patterns are opportunities
for us to adjust and to love

Day 339
Blanketed in Love

Chaos can be calmed by love. Self-love.

Deep in the wild and rambunctious nature of drama, malintent, pain, and suffering, there lies a golden thread.

The word sutra in Sanskrit literally means "thread." Yoga sutras offer wisdom which, when read on days when the mind feels like it is falling apart, can bring the mind together.

This golden thread can be threaded into the eye of a needle so that you can quilt your worth into a form of warmth and shelter for your darkest nights. At that point, the generated love will ease suffering for you and for others.

yoga sutras are threads
we can use to quilt clarity

Day 340
Lighter and Loving

Daily spiritual practice melts questions into faith from which we become lighter and more loving. As sufferings ease, we experience pleasantness for longer periods. From this increased peaceful space in our world we see shifts in our energy, our experiences, and our relationships.

Soon, with strength and might of confident wings, our dreams become tickets to ride. We are gifted the opportunity to fly toward our destiny. Our flight-path in life expands. Soaring through sky, we dance with grace, possibility, abundance, and gratitude.

All of creation, one energy, one love, interconnected—we are it.

Can you see it? Can you feel it from within?

The tools are available: yoga, meditation, yoga sutras, malas and mantras, to name a few. Lose your attachments, close your eyes, and move into the feeling body.

we are all vessels for more and more love—
love never ends

Day 341
I Am River

The river of more-than-enough-ness invites us to bring our kayak or canoe and paddle to places we could never get to on foot. To see wildlife on the riverbanks that can only be seen from the river. To feel nature untouched. If we stay on it for a long time, the river of enough-ness flows into the lake of love, the sea of life, and the oceanic heart. That is the power of the source of the statement, I am.

more than enough is
more than a destination

Day 342
Free Will

Our emotions are a resource. We have free will, at every moment, to choose how we want to think, act, and feel.

Since I began teaching yoga, one of the core practices of my teachings has been to guide and facilitate people to create space and self-regulate so they can change their emotional states at will—to practice being less a piece of creation and more a brilliant creator in and of life.

choice is always yours
you're the boss

Day 343
Seeking

When a relationship sours, we often fail to see how wonderful we are. Discovering even the tiniest part we played in hiding our light from ourselves and others, therefore diminishing our power and capacity to love, is the deepest relationship work a person can do.

discovery is a gamechanger

Day 344
Detachment as Love

Being at peace requires active detachment. When we are in that mode we can see the world doesn't change from crisis, rather it changes in the awareness of people. This goes for a monumental national tragedy and follows the same law for a crisis between two people. Too often we get involved and entangled without detaching. We then have no awareness of desired outcomes or how the messiness will manifest within us. We reach out to others and have perspective around their situations yet find it difficult to apply when we are in a similar situation.

What would it feel like to turn what you offer others you want to help and bring that compassion to yourself?

If relationships are mirrors, what sparks emotion in you about another? Could this be a lesson for your growth now?

our love supply is infinite

Day 345
Preparation

Change is going to take place no matter what. The uncertainty is whether you will make progress when change occurs.

Preparedness for change and progress comes through practice, through being as close to peace as possible so change flows. Progress is a natural branch from that flow.

change + preparedness = progress

Day 346
Comfort Quotes

One of my favourite quotes is from the Greek tragedian, Aeschylus: "Even in our sleep, pain which we cannot forget falls drop by drop upon the heart until, in our own despair, against our will, comes wisdom through the awful grace of God."

That quote comforted me through dark hours in my own life. It reminds me that wisdom is what will rescue me, as well as reward me, for my efforts—and I will grow into a better person from things I've been through.

What can you extract from your darkest days?

Can you use it, if needed, when you have another dark time?

we grow wiser from what we have been
through, no matter how dark the stain

Day 347
Seasons of Love

Our world is weary and grieving, and hearts are heavy with the stress of our global challenges. Yet, as each year ends in the Western world, the messages which flow in at Christmas and of Christmas are poignant.

While Christmas means nothing if we allow it to mean nothing, it means everything if we allow it to be a message from our source, universe, God (love), or whatever your word for destiny is. It is a message that miracles happen. It is a reminder that love solves all problems. It is an affirmation that each of us can give birth to a better version of ourselves. This message provides comfort: none of us are unaccompanied in our efforts to make the world a healed and pleasant place.

the seasons bring messages from which
we can make meaning,
then bring that meaning to life

Day 348
Innate Potentiality

The highest tenets of life and love originate in a plethora of values, including awareness, compassion, empathy, creativity, security, self-esteem, and inner growth. Those values are always within, side by side with a thousand other golden attributes. It's just that our minds wander and skip over them. You can learn to organize your mind so anything you wish for happens.

we are more than our thoughts
we are powerful beyond measure

Day 349
Silence

Meet yourself inside. Take a tour of your values and be impressed by them. Take them out for a stroll. Appreciate them. Then sit with them in quiet and let your awareness settle into pure simplicity: true meditation.

At some point, you will see that everything is created out of nothing, and that nothing is everything.

In that space of calm and clarity, affirm you have nowhere to get to; confirm you are already here.

presence is silence

Day 350
Travel Light

Our thoughts and words become our reality. We create rules and laws for our lives based on our limiting beliefs. If a person says they are clumsy, didn't enjoy gym at school, and professes to be uncoordinated, not only have they heard it from somewhere or someone in their past, they have now made it a reality in their present, so much so that opportunities are missed. Something as magical as dancing at a friend's wedding is never experienced because of an "I'm sorry, I don't dance."

The power our beliefs have over us is profound. In this can you see we are suffering our past and our memories only? Life happens in the present moment, your life is happening right now.

Take a look at some of your strongest negative beliefs: fear of water… can't sing… don't like someone or something. Take a look at some not-so-negative, yet rigid beliefs: need eight hours sleep… must have dessert after dinner… mustn't eat breakfast for supper. Where did these come from? Do you know these things for sure or did culture condition you into them? You can write a list of all the cultural, past, negative, or ancestral thoughts and choose to no longer carry them. Perhaps they have served their purpose and now is for you to serve yours.

when we change our thoughts
we change our lives—be kind

Day 351
Validity

The next time a negative thought shows up, acknowledge it, then evaluate: is it a fact or something I created? Consciously breathe with the thoughts and notice how they make your body feel. Challenge it with a positive action. You cannot control what has already happened or its origin. You can choose what you do in this moment. Decide if you will let it go or keep carrying it with you.

take a few deep breaths and repeat
"I am not my thoughts"

Day 352
Gratitude Attitude

Beauty is everywhere, our awareness fades in the daily rush. Take a moment. Appreciate your surroundings. Cultivate gratitude beginning with what's closest to your body and then expanding gratitude for what is in the room, then the world. Gratitude, like grace, is all around us.

when you see beauty, appreciate it—
express gratitude

Day 353
Nourishment

Surround yourself with nature. Consume foods that resonate with your knowledge of high-quality and less processed. As you embrace the eight limbs, bring your life practices together into a culmination of purity. Include the way you eat your food—mindfully—with the same grace, gratitude, and consideration as you choose the food.

enlightenment includes all aspects
of our lifestyles

Day 354
Samadhi Unfolding

Be not afraid of putting it all together, samadhi. As the final attainment to being, you will maintain your individuality, and how you put it all together will be slightly different than that of another student. As the eight limbs come together in one practice, be the unfolding. Be boldly brave and courageous to shine the light you know is within you.

approach life as a practice
with openness and fearlessness

Day 355
Lifeforce Energy

As you consume pure water, picture it flushing out toxicity. Be the mountain and let the water you drink be the glacial stream. Mindfully focus on the value of this lifegiving elixir.

Take this element seriously, and revere it, be grateful for its presence. Water, like breath, is prana, a lifeforce energy.

existence is miraculous
every breath and every sip is precious

Day 356
Vibe Kind

Giving without expecting anything in return shifts our energy of scarcity to abundance. As we embody all eight limbs, our practice of kindness—and random acts of kindness—can connect us to the intricate web of existence, omnipresence. Kind acts can change lives. Trusting beyond the five senses as to how far the ripple effect of kindness can reach allows us to bathe in the mystery and anonymity of higher consciousness—a profound, private reward.

acts of kindness vibrate love
and compassion from your heart
into the heart of the world—
the same heart beating in your chest

Day 351
Yogis

There's a kind of idea yoga teachers and practitioners who are always zen, chill, graceful, hippie, and happy. Yoga teachers are human beings: the single mom getting two kids out in the morning; the project engineer who has been on-site for two weeks; the bus driver; the grandma; the retail clerk; the police officer; the entrepreneur.

Teaching yoga is absolutely a treasure.

No matter what has happened or is happening in the life of a yoga teacher, good teachers leave it at the door of the studio. Because we have practiced for a long time, we can mirror to others our humanness in all its chaotic glory.

Students come into class wanting headstands, one-legged poses, and the splits. Sometimes we want to say: teaching you to focus on your breath is literally the hardest and most important thing. You don't need fancy poses for a strong yoga practice; you need basic building blocks and your breath. Sometimes the simplest classes are the most challenging.

yoga is a breathing practice, breathing
through the challenge of a pose is yoga

Day 358
Intuitively Teaching

Intuition is a real thing. When it speaks as I teach yoga, I trust it and go with it. These are the greatest classes I recall; they've offered the most value through an epiphany or the achievement and recognition of deep calm for the whole group. There is a palpable energy in all classes, especially at the end of a class that has honoured the collective breath. Sometimes, for me, the whole practice happens at the end, in those moments of calm and clarity.

trust your intuition
it is your best instructor

Day 359
Persistent Effort

When experiencing the culmination of all eight limbs, manifestation will be instant. In samadhi we experience bliss, ecstasy, and oneness. Samadhi vibration, or frequency of our energy, is a natural magnet through which we can manifest our future highest potential selves. Samadhi is impermanent, thus, consistent effort in the two directions inward and outward is required for progress.

we create conditions for transformative
insight to manifest in our experiences

Day 360
Beyond Binds

Fear and worry create a wall between us and what we would like to have or be. That wall is seemingly impenetrable. However, when in the state of samadhi there is no wall. There are no barriers because there is no fear or worry.

The illusion that the five senses are reality has been lifted, like a veil, from our view. We are.

the journey to the state of samadhi
is a quest of epic wonder

Day 361
Embodied Bliss

Mostly a thing of the past: a silent voice. No longer bound by the trappings of judgment and fear, you become a present participant in life… childlike.

In this pure, sacred state, you respond to others with such grace that they are affected immediately by your energy.

the eight limbs of yoga are
gifts given through practice…
you are the jewel in the lotus

Day 362
Courageous Action

If we seek samadhi, we will not find it. Samadhi comes to us as a result of practice and grace. We begin our journey with awareness, and we accumulate compassion along the way. The process as we continue to gather sacred attributes, naturally includes a letting go of those which are not sacred, which do not serve us. Sacrifice is an essential part of the process.

true pleasure is derived
from grace and sacrifice

Day 363
Forging On

Sometimes, people can get caught up in a false samadhi. This is where a person will get a pleasurable, seemingly transcendent moment from an imposter such as drugs, alcohol, overeating, compulsive shopping, gambling, or gaming.

These conflict with reality and bring about lower lows because they create karmic debt. The more highs we experience, the lower the contrasting low.

We are designed to weather great storms, and we can break these karmic patterns. Some things are not as good as they seem, and nothing feels as complete as living a purpose-driven dream.

we are susceptible to false pleasure.
have compassion and forge ahead
in pursuit of your dreams

Day 364
We Arrive Before We Depart

When we truly realize we are not of this world—just a visitor in a vessel called a body—our spirit can live in liberation and guide others. It is a mind-boggling concept, and once attained, it is pure bliss. Freedom and liberation is to be in this world and not of this world. Higher consciousness is a greater sense of purpose and pleasantness serving a higher good.

Our humanness will ebb and flow, of course. With consistent practice, the wondrous knowledge will remain with us and we will have the tools to quickly regain our footing.

we are human, we are spirit,
and we are here to serve

Day 365
Full Circle

The practice of the eight limbs of yoga is a sacred system gifted us by Patañjali. The greatest gift one can receive: freedom from cultural conditioning, from fear, from boasting, from dissatisfaction, and competition.

Even if all of our practices do not reach the point of samadhi, the benefits of practice bless us in myriad ways. We are healthier; we are happier; we are blissful, content, carefree, and caring. Ecstasy comes to some. It will not come to you if chased. Simply go about your loving life practices in peace. It is then you will find presence.

to travel in the world of yoga, there are
many paths which all lead you
to your magnificent heart

All The Love. All The Days.

A perpetual calendar is a wonderful circle of never-ending-ness. We move cyclically as planets, oceans, suns, and moons. Uninhibited, connected, and creating without concern about beginning and end. Our strength, one-mindedness, and elegance is always process and always grace.

Growth is painful—a pain that is ever so natural—and you can handle hard things. As you grow, cycling through again and again, always meet whatever is arising with loving kindness and compassion. Forgive yourself. Loving who you are is a constant garden to be tended infinitely as every moment is impermanent. Humans are designed to love fearlessly and abundantly.

The source of love is infinite, without beginning and without end, as symbolized by the Japanese enso.

When you fall into old patterns, view them as the universe speaking to you through those patterns. Remember your divinity. You are perfectly imperfect for a reason: to experience life and grow. Life, like yoga, is a practice—not perfect. Don't take things seriously or personally. Breathing through the challenges of life and breathing through the challenge of the asana, is yoga. You are love and you are loved.

The love we possess allows us access to become powerful beyond measure. Such love is unmeasurable. Your breath is the bridge from the physical to the spiritual world. Your breath is always there, like a best friend.

Begin Again

The beauty of a revolving 365 practice without a year or date is timeless—as are you, as is the practice of yoga. Love, life, yoga, goes on, beyond the mat, beyond the years, ageless, limitless, and pure potentiality to renew, restore, forgive, become all you dream to be and so much more. Love never ends, so begin this cycle again and again, yoga teacher Pattabhi Jois said: "Keep going, there is more."

We are as layers of an onion. We peel them back, layer after layer, petal after petal. You keep on keeping on; there is no core.

May you commit to begin again, to practice remembering each day—a commitment to your heart, reinspired not only by the printed page, perhaps also by any notes or doodles you made on those pages.

We are all writing our heart's whispers and singing the song of our connected soul.

And when you are ready to peel back more layers, consider purchasing the Deeper Days Companion Journal, available here: ingeniumbooks.com/DeeperDaysJournal

Much love, Andrea

Acknowledgements

Thank you Jeff Godin. Your computer support, compiling my writings from cases of floppy discs, broken laptops, Word documents and on hard drives has been and continues to be the magic behind my dream of writing books.

Thank you to Boni (John is in the background here too, silent, brilliant, supportive) at Ingenium Books who literally and continually breathes life into my ideas, supporting my dreams. You are light, essential to my visionary soul. Thank you for talking me through tears, guiding me beyond my years and not leaving me when I thought I failed edits horribly.

Thank you to Melissa Loft for your shoulder to lean and cry on, your heart for understanding the highs and lows of following a dream, and for your constant presence in my life. My books would not be written without your positivity shining through any self doubts I toss your way.

Thank you Jessica Bell for following your heart and touching mine with your cover designs.

Thank you to my latest editor who bit off a lot of yoga chew. May we all have deeper days and ease of heart ways because of your work behind my daily 2278 practices collection that we narrowed down to 365.

To my readers. Our hearts are joined. I bow deeply and thank you kindly.

To those I love, you know I do, you know first-hand my practice to always tell you, mail you and leave things on your doorsteps.

There is no yoga without relationships. I thank my mediation teachers, my reiki master teachers, my Ashtanga teacher, my Hatha teacher, my reconnective healing teacher and doctor, my NLP teacher and my Zen Buddhist teacher.

I thank the men who let me love them intimately, deeply. I learned and loved each moment with you.

Without knowing my grandparents, especially my four grandmothers, I may not have known I could be this strong.

About the Author

Andrea L. Wehlann is a certified Hatha Yoga teacher and owns and operates the Ganga Moon Yoga Studio in Beamsville, Ontario, Canada. With a BA in psychology from Brock University and a social services diploma from Niagara College, Andrea's work in the social services field, as well as a Reiki Master, Brazilian Jiu Jitsu, Chi Kung, Feng Shui, and meditation practitioner round out her experience. She's the author of two books for women: *Deeper Days* is her second, which follows the full-length poetry collection, *No Matter How Dark The Stain: Poems and Inspiration for the Woman in Pain* (Ingenium Books, 2021).

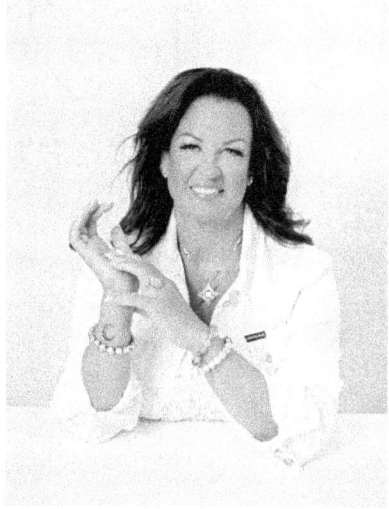

Her dedication to spiritual healing comes from overcoming childhood, mental, physical, and emotional abuse, surviving rape and sexual assault, miscarriages and infant loss—personal experiences that make her an effective healer today.

Andrea has received the Editor's Choice Award for Outstanding Achievement in Poetry by The National Library of Poetry (Canada), Honourable Mention from Iliad Press, and a Poet of Merit Award. Her poetry has been published in The Brock Press Literary Supplement, The 1996 Blue Ribbon Collection, Portraits of Life published by the National Library of Poetry and the International Society of Poets, and Another Nobody: A Tribute to the Homeless by Niagara's Poets. Andrea was a distinguished member of the International Society of Poets for more than seven years and has in the past been a member of The Canadian Theosophical Society. She's been featured in publications like Niagara Life Magazine.

The Deeper Days Habit Tracker

Sustain your daily practice through *Deeper Days*
with this habit tracker and reflection sheet.

Download your free tracker at
ingeniumbooks.com/deeperdaystracker

www.ingramcontent.com/pod-product-compliance
Lightning Source LLC
Chambersburg PA
CBHW022042020426
42335CB00012B/508